Advances in Acne Management

Editors

JAMES Q. DEL ROSSO

JOSHUA A. ZEICHNER

DERMATOLOGIC CLINICS

www.derm.theclinics.com

Consulting Editor
BRUCE H. THIERS

April 2016 • Volume 34 • Number 2

ELSEVIER

1600 John F. Kennedy Boulevard • Suite 1800 • Philadelphia, Pennsylvania, 19103-2899

http://www.theclinics.com

DERMATOLOGIC CLINICS Volume 34, Number 2
April 2016 ISSN 0733-8635, ISBN-13: 978-0-323-41752-5

Editor: Jessica McCool
Developmental Editor: Alison Swety

Dermatologic Clinics (ISSN 0733-8635) is published quarterly by Elsevier Inc., 360 Park Avenue South, New York, NY 10010-1710. Months of publication are January, April, July, and October. Business and editorial offices: 1600 John F. Kennedy Blvd., Suite 1800, Philadelphia, PA 19103-2899. Customer service office: 11830 Westline Drive, St. Louis, MO 63146. Periodicals postage paid at New York, NY, and additional mailing offices. Subscription prices are USD 370.00 per year for US individuals, USD 618.00 per year for US institutions, USD 425.00 per year for Canadian individuals, USD 754.00 per year for Canadian institutions, USD 495.00 per year for international individuals, USD 754.00 per year for international institutions, USD 100.00 per year for US students/residents, and USD 240.00 per year for Canadian and international students/residents. International air speed delivery is included in all *Clinics* subscription prices. All prices are subject to change without notice. **POSTMASTER:** Send address changes to *Dermatologic Clinics*, Elsevier Health Sciences Division, Subscription Customer Service, 3251 Riverport Lane, Maryland Heights, MO 63043. **Customer Service: 1-800-654-2452 (U.S. and Canada); 314-447-8871 (outside U.S. and Canada). Fax: 314-447-8029. E-mail: journalscustomerservice-usa@elsevier.com (for print support); journalsonlinesupport-usa@elsevier.com (for online support).**

Reprints. For copies of 100 or more, of articles in this publication, please contact the Commercial Reprints Department, Elsevier Inc., 360 Park Avenue South, New York, New York 10010-1710. Tel.: 212-633-3874; Fax: 212-633-3820; Email: reprints@elsevier.com.

The *Dermatologic Clinics* is covered in *MEDLINE/PubMed (Index Medicus)*, *Current Contents/Clinical Medicine*, *Excerpta Medica*, *Chemical Abstracts*, and *ISI/BIOMED*.

Contributors

CONSULTING EDITOR

BRUCE H. THIERS, MD
Professor and Chairman, Department of
Dermatology and Dermatologic Surgery,
Medical University of South Carolina,
Charleston, South Carolina

EDITORS

JAMES Q. DEL ROSSO, DO
Adjunct Clinical Professor, Dermatology, Touro
University Nevada, Henderson, Nevada; Lakes
Dermatology, Las Vegas, Nevada

JOSHUA A. ZEICHNER, MD
Assistant Professor, Department of
Dermatology, Icahn School of Medicine at
Mount Sinai, New York, New York

AUTHORS

SANWARJIT BOYAL, BMSc
Research Assistant, Windsor Clinical Research
Inc, Windsor, Ontario, Canada

JAMES Q. DEL ROSSO, DO
Adjunct Clinical Professor, Dermatology, Touro
University Nevada, Henderson, Nevada; Lakes
Dermatology, Las Vegas, Nevada

KARISHMA DESAI, BMSc
Department of Medicine, Schulich School of
Medicine and Dentistry, Western University,
Windsor, Ontario, Canada

DOUGLAS FIFE, MD
Surgical Dermatology and Laser Center, Las
Vegas, Nevada

JULIE C. HARPER, MD
The Dermatology and Skin Care Center of
Birmingham, Birmingham, Alabama

SANJA KNEZEVIC, BSc
Department of Medicine, Schulich School of
Medicine and Dentistry, Western University,
Windsor, Ontario, Canada

ANDREW C. KRAKOWSKI, MD
Assistant Clinical Professor, Division of
Pediatric and Adolescent Dermatology, Rady
Children's Hospital, San Diego, California;
DermOne, LLC, West Conshohocken,
Pennsylvania

ALISON M. LAYTON, MB ChB, FRCP (UK)
Department of Dermatology, Harrogate and
District NHS Foundation Trust, Harrogate,
North Yorkshire, United Kingdom

JACQUELYN LEVIN, DO, FAOCD
Largo Medical Center, Dermatology Division,
Largo, Florida

ANGELA MACRI, DO
Center for Clinical and Cosmetic Research,
Aventura, Florida

LIDIA MAROÑAS-JIMÉNEZ, MD
Department of Dermatology, Hospital
Universitario 12 de Octubre, Medical School,
Universidad Complutense, Institute i+12,
Madrid, Spain

MORGAN McCARTY, DO
Assistant Clinical Professor Dermatology,
Department of Dermatology; Baylor
Scott & White Clinical Assistant Professor,
Scott & White Healthcare, Temple, Texas

MARK S. NESTOR, MD, PhD
Center for Clinical and Cosmetic Research;
Center for Cosmetic Enhancement Director,
Aventura, Florida; Department of Dermatology
and Cutaneous Surgery, Department of
Surgery, Division of Plastic Surgery, University
of Miami Miller School of Medicine, Miami,
Florida

HYUNHEE PARK, DO
Dermatology Resident, Department of
Dermatology, Larkin Community Hospital/
NSU-COM, Margate, Florida

NANETTE SILVERBERG, MD
Clinical Professor of Dermatology and
Pediatrics; Director, Pediatric and Adolescent
Dermatology; Chief, Pediatric Dermatology,

Icahn School of Medicine at Mount Sinai;
Mount Sinai St. Luke's Roosevelt Hospital
Center, New York, New York

STANLEY SKOPIT, DO, MSE, FAOCD
Program Director, Dermatology Residency
Program, Larkin Community Hospital/
NSU-COM, Margate, Florida

NICOLE SWENSON, DO
Center for Clinical and Cosmetic Research,
Aventura, Florida

JERRY TAN, MD, FRCPC
Adjunct Professor of Dermatology, Faculty of
Medicine, Schulich School of Medicine and
Dentistry, Western University; Dermatologist,
Windsor Clinical Research Inc, Windsor,
Ontario, Canada

JOSHUA A. ZEICHNER, MD
Assistant Professor, Department of
Dermatology, Icahn School of Medicine at
Mount Sinai, New York, New York

Contents

The Internet provides both education and miseducation for acne patients. Although some sites provide disease background information and objective treatment guidance, support networks, and research findings, others may seem to be objective on the surface, but are in reality run by untrained, self-proclaimed experts or are promotional in nature. Providers must be aware of the potential benefits and pitfalls the Internet provides for those suffering with acne.

Patients often perceive the cause of their acne to be related to a lack of proper cleansing, therefore many patients attempt to treat their acne either alone or with prescription therapy by frequent aggressive cleansing with harsh cleansing agents. Altered epidermal barrier function, inflammation, and *Propionibacterium acnes* are related to acne vulgaris (AV) pathophysiology; proper cleansing can favorably modulate the development of AV. The available clinical studies support gentle cleansing in AV by showing the ability to contribute to improving AV lesion counts and severity and minimizing the irritation seen with topical AV therapies such as retinoids and BP.

Acne represents the most common inflammatory dermatosis seen worldwide and is the leading reason for seeing a dermatologist. This article provides some tips for managing acne in a safe and effective manner to minimize the physical and psychological scars that can result from acne. Tips include how to optimize available treatment regimens according to the evidence base and target therapy to pathophysiologic factors, while also tailoring treatments to patient expectation and needs. Attention is given to minimizing the emergence of antimicrobial resistance in acne patients and beyond.

Acne vulgaris may be effectively treated with combination oral contraceptive pills (COCs) in women. COCs may be useful in any woman with acne in the absence of known contraindications. When prescribing a COC to a woman who also desires contraception, the risks of the COC are compared with the risks associated with pregnancy. When prescribing a COC to a woman who does not desire contraception, the risks of the COC must be weighed against the risks associated with acne. COCs may take 3 cycles of use to show an effect in acne lesion count reductions.

Antibiotics are commonly used by dermatologists in clinical practice, primarily because of the overall track record of favorable efficacy and safety with the most commonly used agents. During the past decade, increased attention has been given to the problems associated with antibiotic resistance. This article summarizes important principles gleaned from the continued efforts of the Scientific Panel on Antibiotic Use in Dermatology; other groups working diligently in this area, such as the Centers for Disease Control and Prevention and the Canadian Antimicrobial Resistance Alliance; and from the published literature.

Oral isotretinoin is unrivalled in efficacy and remission capability for treatment of acne. In addition to appropriate monitoring and continued vigilance for safety concerns, appropriate dosing to mitigate avoidable dose-dependent adverse effects is the responsibility of prescribers. Low-dose regimens are better tolerated and effective in inducing acne clearance. Although much progress has been made since the advent of isotretinoin, there remain many unanswered questions regarding optimization to maximize response while minimizing the potential for avoidable adverse events. The ongoing availability of isotretinoin is imperative to patients with acne, their caregivers, and physicians.

Acne vulgaris, a disorder of the pilosebaceous unit, is one of the most commonly encountered conditions in dermatology practice. Effective treatment of acne vulgaris is important in that it can prevent psychosocial distress and physical scarring. Systemic therapeutic options are available for moderate to severe acne. It is imperative that the safe and effective treatment revolves around the health care provider's familiarity of side effects of various treatments. In this article, the side effects and monitoring guide for the most commonly prescribed systemic agents for acne vulgaris are reviewed.

Acne vulgaris presenting from birth to preadolescence can be confusing to diagnose and even more challenging to evaluate and manage. The differential diagnosis of acne varies by age and, in some cases (especially when it presents in midchildhood), deserves a thorough evaluation to rule out underlying systemic abnormalities. Acne management strategies, including factors affecting adherence to the treatment regimen, may be influenced by the patient's age. This article presents an overview of the clinical presentations of acne by age and our approach to evaluation and management of this common condition.

Acne vulgaris alters the normal skin physiology, impairing stratum corneum and transepidermal water loss. A male's normal skin physiologic state is different than a female's and may have implications when choosing treatment when the skin is altered in a disease state. Transepidermal water loss, pH, and sebum production are different between the sexes. Several underlying conditions present in male acne patients at several ages that may require a more in-depth evaluation. As knowledge of the pathogenesis of acne expands, the differences in skin physiology between the sexes may alter the manner in which male patients with acne medications are approached.

The prevalence and emotional impact of acne scarring are underestimated by the medical community. Dermatology providers should be able to evaluate the acne scar patient and discuss treatment options. Important aspects of the patient history include current treatments, prior acne scar procedures, and the patient's goals for treatment. During the physical examination, the scars are assessed and classified by scar morphology and overall severity of scarring. Finally, a treatment plan is developed in which the most appropriate procedures are matched with the scars that will work the best. Helping the patient understand likely expectations for improvement will increase overall satisfaction.

Treatment options for acne vulgaris are enhanced by laser and light therapy. Both visible and laser light are effective treatments for acne. Visible light and many lasers target Propionibacterium acnes porphyrins while others act as anti-inflammatory mediators or reduce sebaceous gland activity. Compared with topical and systemic therapies, laser and light therapies have few if any side effects and appear to be safe during pregnancy. If patients prefer at home light treatments, several devices are currently available and have been shown to have efficacy. Ultimately, combining laser and light with topical therapy may well become the mainstay of acne treatment.

Acne vulgaris (AV) is considered a straightforward diagnosis made clinically without specific diagnostic testing. However, certain disorders may simulate AV, such as multiple small epidermal cysts or deep milia, multiple osteoma cutis, multiple small adnexal neoplasms, and follicular and/or infections characterized by multiple small papules and/or pustules such as gram-positive folliculitis, gram-negative folliculitis, *Malassezia* folliculitis, keratosis pilaris, and flat warts. This can lead to an erroneous diagnosis and improper management. Acneiform eruptions, often associated with ingestion of certain drugs and chemicals, can confound the clinician regarding AV diagnosis. This article presents an interesting case that was originally misdiagnosed as AV.

DERMATOLOGIC CLINICS

Preface
Face to Face with Acne in 2016 and Beyond

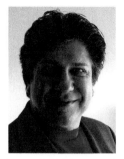 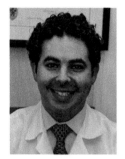

James Q. Del Rosso, DO   Joshua A. Zeichner, MD

Editors

What is not new is that acne vulgaris (AV) continues to be the most common skin disease encountered in outpatient dermatology practice in the United States. What is new are some of the modern-day challenges clinicians face in managing their patients with AV. One major current challenge is self-management by patients via information sources and product offerings on the Internet, which frequently lead to delays in seeking appropriate care and poor adherence. This often results in unfortunate sequelae such as facial and truncal scarring and persistent dyspigmentation. Other practical challenges include cost factors and difficulties achieving medication access due to complicated and idiosyncratic systems put in place by third-party payors. On a daily basis, clinicians and their office staff battle through these and other challenges when trying to optimally treat their patients with AV.

Beyond the aforementioned practical and logistical challenges, the clinician must keep abreast of current information on the pathophysiology of AV, proper skin care, topical and systemic therapies, physical modality options, and adverse reactions. To add, it is very important for clinicians to consider the potential clinical relevance of bacterial resistance to antibiotics when prescribing these agents, especially as management of AV is typically a prolonged process. It is important for all clinicians to maintain an open mind as new information emerges by evaluating the quality and accuracy of the information and determining if it may be relevant to improving treatment outcomes in their patients with AV.

In this issue of *Dermatologic Clinics*, we have put together a collection of articles that addresses a broad range of topics that are very relevant to clinicians who treat patients with AV. Authors were selected based on their areas of interest; knowledge and clinical expertise; and a desire to include some "newer names" into the publication arena on AV. It is our hope that you find the articles in this issue enlightening academically and valuable clinically.

James Q. Del Rosso, DO
Dermatology
Touro University Nevada
Henderson, NV, USA

Lakes Dermatology
8861 West Sahara Avenue
Suite 290
Las Vegas, NV 89117, USA

Joshua A. Zeichner, MD
Icahn School of Medicine at Mount Sinai
64 East 86 Street, Apartment 3B
New York, NY 10028, USA

E-mail addresses:
jqdelrosso@yahoo.com (J.Q. Del Rosso)
Joshua.Zeichner@mountsinai.org (J.A. Zeichner)

Dermatol Clin 34 (2016) ix
http://dx.doi.org/10.1016/j.det.2016.01.001
0733-8635/16/$ – see front matter © 2016 Published by Elsevier Inc.

Acne and the Internet

Joshua A. Zeichner, MD[a],*, James Q. Del Rosso, DO[b]

KEYWORDS

• Acne • Internet • Google • Website • Patient education

KEY POINTS

- Patients commonly search for medical information, particularly about acne, on the Internet.
- Although there is much useful information about acne on the Internet, there is also a lot of misinformation and promotional information masquerading as education.
- Providers must be aware of reliable Internet resources so they can refer interested patients for more information on acne or other disease states.

INTRODUCTION

The Internet has emerged as the primary resource for almost all daily activities, ranging from shopping to education. In the health care space, online information continues to increase. One study from 2012 showed that 70% of adults used the Internet as their initial source of health information.[1] Adolescents especially have been found to prefer seeking out health care information from the Internet. In fact, that may be the adolescent patient's only source of health information.[2] The Internet provides users with access to disease-specific symptoms and treatments, the ability to connect with others for advice and support, and knowledge of up-to-date research, breakthroughs, and clinical trials. Although Internet access is widely available, there is much miseducation as not everything published online is reliable. The Internet affects the doctor–patient relationship, because many patients come to the office armed with what may or may not be correct information. The doctor must be aware of this when engaging patients. Treatment recommendations should include not only prescription therapies, but also referrals to reliable online resources for interested patients.

Acne vulgaris affects an estimated 40 million Americans each year, the majority of whom are adolescents and teenagers.[3] Given this younger, Internet-savvy demographic, it is not surprising that many patients are using the web as a source for information on acne. Since 2008, Internet searches for the keyword "acne" have continued to increase and are greater than that of other skin diseases. Interestingly, search volume for the term "acne" peaks over the weekend, with a relative lull during the week. It is thought that this trend is attributable to younger people being busy with school during the week and having more free time during the weekends.[4]

The Global Burden of Disease 2010 project evaluated the impact of 291 diseases, including those of the skin, on quality of life.[5] It has been shown that the volume of disease search terms on Google strongly correlates to the burden of the disease according to the Global Burden of Disease 2010 data.[6] Of the 15 skin diseases included in the Global Burden of Disease 2010 data, acne received the highest Internet search interest, followed closely only by herpes.[6] Acne has been shown to affect quality of life as much as other significant, chronic diseases such as severe asthma, epilepsy, and diabetes.[7] Internet search term data reflects this as well. In 2013, the term "acne" was more searched for on Google than even the term "diabetes."[4]

WHAT IS OUT THERE

Acne patients are actively seeking out information online. However, there is no regulation over the quality or accuracy of what they are reading. Available online resources may be broadly divided into

---

[a] Department of Dermatology, Icahn School of Medicine at Mount Sinai, 5 East 98 Street, 5th Floor, New York, NY 10029, USA; [b] Dermatology, Touro University Nevada, 874 American Pacific Drive, Henderson, NV 89014, USA

* Corresponding author.
E-mail address: joshua.zeichner@mountsinai.org

Dermatol Clin 34 (2016) 129–132
http://dx.doi.org/10.1016/j.det.2015.12.001

4 different categories: (1) educational websites from well-respected organizations, (2) promotional websites, (3) independent websites from self-proclaimed experts, and (4) social media websites. It is important to understand the differences between these types of websites, the information they provide, and the potential ramifications they can have on patients and the doctor–patient relationship.

Educational Websites from Well-respected Organizations

Many academic centers, government institutions, professional organizations, and health journals provide publicly available health information. Using the term "acne" in a Google search yields the following sites among the top of search list: The American Academy of Dermatology (AAD), Medline Plus from the US National Library of Medicine, and the National Institute of Arthritis and Musculoskeletal and Skin Diseases, a division of the National Institutes of Health. Some academic centers and hospitals also provide web-based health information. The most popular of these sites include the Mayo Clinic and Johns Hopkins Medicine. Each of these sites provides unbiased, educational information on the causes, clinical presentation, and potential therapies for acne. They can all be considered high-quality, reliable resources for patients (**Table 1**).

The AAD provides extensive public education materials on its own website and should be considered a go-to referral resource for patients. Specifically, it contains a "Derm A to Z" section with well-written articles and a video series that cover skin diseases as well as health and beauty. The public site content is regularly reviewed by the academy's Public Education Committee to ensure that information is medically accurate, up to date, and delivers key messages that dermatologists want their patients and the public to know.

Articles from health and lifestyle magazines are commonly available online in addition to print. Although most of the content of these articles has undergone a fact checking process, it cannot be universally assumed. Many articles feature quotes from board-certified dermatologists, which adds credibility to articles; however, quality varies from 1 publication to another. WebMD is one example of a high-quality magazine that offers education on par with some of the previously mentioned websites.

Promotional Websites

Promotional websites may not be easily identified. What seems at first to be solely an educational resource may in fact be a façade designed to sell an acne or skin care treatment. Professional marketers, salesmen, and website designers purposefully create content or chat boards to engage users, who are ultimately directed to make some sort of purchase. These sites are the online equivalent to paid promotional "advertorials" seen in print magazines. Here, educational content that mimics an unpaid article is created. However, the entire page has a focused, biased direction and is in fact a paid advertisement. Although some useful information may be obtained from sites like this, it is important to understand that the root of the website is based on selling a skin care regimen.

Independent Websites from Self-proclaimed Authorities

Creating a website is as easy as purchasing a domain name and registering with a host server, many of which provide easy-to-use site-building software. Armed with a credit card, a technologically savvy person can create a blog portraying him or herself under any persona and post whatever he or she likes. Although some blogs are quite popular, with thousands of subscribers, popularity does not equal accuracy. Most blogs narrate personal experiences and opinions (positive or negative), which may or may not be based on fact. Some contain useful information, with references to medical literature or consultations with dermatologists. However, others may have undisclosed, ulterior motives. Many independent bloggers may have financial conflicts with products being reviewed. Others may make unsubstantiated,

Table 1 Reliable online acne resources	
AAD: Derm A to Z	www.aad.org/dermatology-a-to-z/diseases-and-treatments/a—d/acne
Medline Plus	www.nlm.nih.gov/medlineplus/acne.html
NIAMS	www.niams.nih.gov/Health_Info/Acne/
Mayo Clinic	www.mayoclinic.org/diseases-conditions/acne/basics/definition/con-20020580
WebMD	www.webmd.com/skin-problems-and-treatments/acne/
E-medicine: Medscape	http://emedicine.medscape.com/article/1069804-overview

uneducated claims that dermatologists may feel are closer to fiction than fact. In this way, some blogs can be more harmful than helpful. By offering specific treatment advice to readers, they may delay patients in seeking professional care or even question professional advice. No professional degree is necessary to become a blogger or to gain a popular following. Ultimately, it is important to understand that a blogger offering acne advice may be a self-proclaimed expert, rather than a formally educated one.

Social Media

Millions of users visit social media sites around the world every day. They allow individuals or groups to create profiles and engage other users by sharing messages, photos, and videos. Popular sites include Facebook, Twitter, LinkedIn, YouTube, and Instagram. They have become popular outlets for patients to interact with each other and discuss specific health concerns.[8] Twitter is a site in which users write short, 140 character posts that may include links or photos. It is estimated that twitter engages 300 million monthly users, with 500 million tweets sent every day. Moreover, 80% of users access it with a mobile device.[9] Facebook is a site in which users or organizations create a profile page on which "status updates" may be posted, with text, photos, and videos. Facebook's 2015 second quarter report estimated 1.49 billion monthly active users, a 13% increase from the previous year. The majority of users (1.31 billion) are engaging on a mobile device.[10]

These sites are being recognized as a useful tool by professional health care communities. A recent study published in *JAMA Dermatology* reported an increase in the use of social media websites by medical journals, professional dermatology organizations, and patient-centered dermatology organizations.[11] The *Journal of the American Academy of Dermatology* and *DermTimes* were reported to be the leading dermatology publications on social media. The dermRounds Dermatology network was the sited example of a professional organization using both Facebook and Twitter. The most popular patient-centered organizations included the Skin Cancer Foundation, DermaTalk, and the National Psoriasis Foundation. Social media offers a way to extend the organizations' reach to dermatology health care professionals and beyond, to the public at large. The online networks have endless potential benefits in driving education in dermatology, providing reliable information from credible sources.

Acne is a particularly popular topic on social media sites. Although posts by professional organizations may be vetted and objective, social media is largely unregulated and more commonly used by patients to discuss personal opinions. As a result, there is potential for much misinformation in this space. One recent study evaluated Twitter posts that contained a key world related to acne (pimple, pimples, zit, zits, and acne). Over a 2-week period, a total of 392,617 tweets were found, 8192 of which were considered high impact, because they were retweeted by other users. Only a minority of the high-impact tweets were about "disease information" (16.9%) and "treatment information" (8.9%). The most common tweets were "personal" (43.1%), about "celebrities" (20.4%), or "education related" (27.1%).[12]

ONLINE DANGERS

With "cybereducation" comes potential danger. The Internet brings access not only to information, but also to medications. When properly prescribed and monitored, drugs like isotretinoin can be used safely. However, without proper supervision, patients can experience potentially serious consequences. A Google search using the term "isotretinoin online" brings with it suggested similar search terms including "isotretinoin online pharmacy," "isotretinoin online India," and "isotretinoin online Canadian pharmacy" (Fig. 1). Links to dozens of online pharmacies are available, where

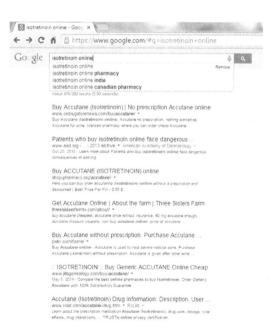

Fig. 1. A Google search using the keywords "isotretinoin online" provides multiple resources to obtain isotretinoin outside of a physician's supervision or compliance with the iPledge Program. (Google and the Google logo are registered trademarks of Google Inc., used with permission.)

the isotretinoin can easily be purchased using a credit card, without a prescription, without participation in the iPledge program, and without a doctor's supervision. Even more worrisome is the accessibility of the drug to women of childbearing potential, who are not necessarily on 2 forms of contraception. In 2007, the US Food and Drug Administration published a press release warning consumers about the dangers of purchasing isotretinoin online.[13] The AAD published a statement echoing the US Food and Drug Administration in 2013, which now lives on the AAD's website.[14] The reality of the situation is that patients determined to obtain the drug independently may be able to do so, because it is difficult to regulate patients and Internet pharmacies. However, in the event that patients come to our practices with isotretinoin obtained through the Internet, we must educate them and urge them to comply with government regulations and iPledge, which US physicians and pharmacies are obliged to comply with as well.

SUMMARY

The Internet brings both pros and cons for our acne patients. Patients with common interests can connect and form support networks. They can become self-educated, but we must be aware that there is much "miseducation." Whether we agree with available online resources or not, the Internet is here to stay. The doctor–patient relationship is evolving with a new generation cybereducated patients. In interacting with our patients, dermatologists must be cognizant of the Internet and social media. As part of our patient education, we must clarify myths and correct misperceptions learned online. Moreover, in addition to treatment, we must also provide reliable online educational resources. There will likely come a day when most dermatologists will be interacting with patients not only in the office, but also actively engaging them in the online space as well.

REFERENCES

1. Prestin A, Vieux SN, Chou WY. Is online health activity alive and well or flatlining? Findings from 10 years of the health information national trends survey. J Health Commun 2015;20(7):790–8.

2. Gray NJ, Klein JD, Noyce PR, et al. Health information-seeking behaviour in adolescence: the place of the internet. Soc Sci Med 2005;60:1467–78.

3. Thiboutot DM. Acne. An overview of clinical research findings. Dermatol Clin 1997;15(1):97–109.

4. Shin HT, Park SW, Lee DY. Relative high interest in acne on the internet: a web-based comparison using google trends. Ann Dermatol 2014;26(5):641–2.

5. Murray CJ, Ezzati M, Flaxman AD, et al. GBD 2010: design, definitions, and metrics. Lancet 2012; 280(9859):2063–6.

6. Whitsitt J, Karimkhani C, Boyers L, et al. Comparing burden of dermatologist disease to search interest on google trends. Dermatol Online J 2015;21(1).

7. Mallon E, Newton JN, Klassen A, et al. The quality of life in acne: a comparison with general medical conditions using generic questionnaires. Br J Dermatol 1999;140(4):672–6.

8. Boyer C. Social media for healthcare makes sense. Front Health Serv Manage 2011;28(2):35–40.

9. Twitter. Learn Twitter. Available at: https://business. twitter.com/basics/learn-twitter. Accessed July 31, 2015.

10. Facebook. Investor Relations. Available at: http:// investor.fb.com/releasedetail.cfm?ReleaseID=924562. Accessed July 21, 2015.

11. Amir M, Sampson BP, Endly D, et al. Social networking sites emerging and essential tools for communication in dermatology. JAMA Dermatol 2014;150(1):56–60.

12. Shive M, Bhatt M, Cantino A, et al. Perspectives on acne: what twitter can teach health care professionals. JAMA Dermatol 2013;149(5):621–2.

13. US Food and Drug Administration. News & Events. Available at: www.fda.gov/NewsEvents/Newsroom/PressAnnouncements/2007/ucm108876.htm. Accessed July 31, 2015.

14. American Academy of Dermatology (AAD). Member to Member Archives. Available at: www.aad.org/members/publications/member-to-member/2013-archive/october-25-2013/patients-who-buy-isotretinoin-online-face-dangerous-consequences. Accessed July 31, 2015.

The Relationship of Proper Skin Cleansing to Pathophysiology, Clinical Benefits, and the Concomitant Use of Prescription Topical Therapies in Patients with Acne Vulgaris

Jacquelyn Levin, DO, FAOCD

KEYWORDS

- Acne vulgaris • OTC products • Surfactants • Skin irritation • Skin barrier function • Sensitive skin
- Retinoids • Benzoyl peroxide

KEY POINTS

- Patients often perceive the cause of their acne to be related to poor hygiene and a lack of proper cleansing, therefore many patients with acne attempt to treat their acne either alone or with prescription therapy by frequent aggressive skin cleansing with harsh cleansing agents.
- Altered epidermal barrier function, inflammation, and *Propionibacterium acnes* are related components to acne vulgaris (AV) pathophysiology; proper cleansing can favorably modulate the development of AV.
- Benzoyl peroxide (BP) and topical retinoid therapy (ie, tretinoin) can adversely alter skin barrier function and cause cutaneous irritation, thus affecting patient tolerability and compliance with AV. Improvements in vehicle technology may mitigate the barrier impairment that may be associated with these therapeutic agents.
- Harsh cleansers, such as true soap and cleansers with high alkaline pH, adversely affect the skin by increasing skin pH, impairing the stratum corneum (SC) permeability barrier function, altering skin bacterial flora, desiccating the SC, increasing erythema, inducing symptoms of subjective irritation, and promoting follicular plugging.
- Combars with an added antibacterial agent do not decrease the amount of *P acnes* on skin and may promote gram-negative folliculitis if there is preferential reduction in commensal gram-positive bacteria. Therefore, true soap and combars are not ideal products to use in most skin diseases, including AV.
- Syndet bars and lipid-free cleansers have the potential to gently cleanse the skin without markedly diminishing epidermal barrier function. This process optimally prepares the SC for the application and absorption of topical therapies while minimizing skin irritation, reducing skin dehydration from prescription therapies, and maintaining the physiologic acid mantle pH of the skin.
- The limited clinical studies available support the benefit of gentle cleansing in AV by showing the ability to contribute to improving AV lesion counts and severity and minimizing the irritation seen with topical AV therapies such as retinoids and BP.

Largo Medical Center, Dermatology Division, 201 14th St SW, Largo, FL 33770, USA
E-mail address: jlevin@hotmail.com

Dermatol Clin 34 (2016) 133–145
http://dx.doi.org/10.1016/j.det.2015.11.001
0733-8635/16/$ – see front matter © 2016 Elsevier Inc. All rights reserved.

INTRODUCTION

Worldwide, acne vulgaris (AV) is one of the skin disorders for which patients most frequently consult a dermatologist.[1] The economic and psychosocial burden of AV is high, and it constitutes the most common reason for dermatologist consultation.[2,3] The direct cost of AV in the United States is estimated to exceed $1 billion per year, with $100 million spent on over-the-counter (OTC) AV products.[3,4]

AV is a polymorphic skin disorder that produces a series of lesions: comedones, cysts, pustules, papules, or nodules. The primary goals of acne therapy are to achieve initial control, maintain therapy to prevent flares, and prevent persistent or permanent sequelae such as scarring. An important aspect of AV management that is often forgotten by physicians is to dispel any myths and misperceptions the patient may have about the cause of their AV, and to develop an appropriate management plan that includes adjunctive OTC products that serve to support their prescription regimen.[4]

Many patients with AV mistakenly think that aggressively cleansing their skin with soap and water several times a day is therapeutic for AV. A survey of patient perceptions of AV showed that 29% of patients thought AV was caused by poor skin hygiene, and 18% thought it was caused by infection, with 61% of patients thinking dirt was an aggravating factor.[5,6] Even among medical students, 25% thought poor facial hygiene was an exacerbating factor.[6] For generations, even physicians thought that successful treatment of AV depended on the degreasing of the skin to an extent that produces desquamation with noticeable peeling.[7] Because of these perceptions, patients tend to cleanse diligently and harshly with the belief that the more cleansing the better.

In the 1980s things started to change and the suggestion was made that inducing visible inflammation and desquamation of the skin was not necessary for acne control.[5,6] Also, it was discovered that the lipid in the follicular reservoir that plays a role in AV pathogenesis cannot likely be reached by harsh soaps and detergents or by frenetic washing; aggressive cleansing with harsh soaps can aggravate AV and, under certain circumstances, cause a detergent-induced acneiform eruption.[8] In addition, over-zealous cleansing can lead to disruption of the epidermal barrier,[9–11] increased transepidermal water loss (TEWL),[9–11] roughened and irritated skin,[10,12] increased bacterial colonization,[12] increased comedonal formation,[8] secondary irritant contact dermatitis,[10] and burning and stinging.[13–15] These negative effects caused by harsh soaps and aggressive cleansing make many prescription topical AV medications less tolerable.[4,16] It is for these reasons that many dermatologists are now recommending gentle cleansers rather than the harsh soaps and cleansers used in the past with the hope of improved patient outcomes and increased compliance.[9]

Although there is a plethora of data on the tolerability and benefits of mild cleansers in other skin disease, such as atopic dermatitis, data are more limited concerning their benefit in AV.[11,17–21]

This article presents and summarizes the available scientific evidence concerning the use of gentle cleansers in AV.

ACNE PATHOGENESIS

The pathogenesis of acne is multifactorial, involving follicular hyperkeratinization leading to (1) comedo formation; (2) hormonal (androgenic) stimulation of the sebaceous glands leading to increased sebaceous gland size and sebum secretion; (3) proliferation of Propionibacterium acnes; and (4) induction of a variety of inflammatory cascades, some triggered in response to P acnes proliferation. These factors are summarized in **Box 1**.[22]

Follicular Wall Barrier Dysfunction

One of the primary events in the pathophysiology of acne is subclinical aberrant follicular wall hyperkeratinization,[23,24] leading to a plugged follicular orifice (microcomedo).[23] There several hypotheses regarding the pathophysiologic mechanism of follicular wall hyperkeratinization seen in acne; however, decreased stratum corneum (SC) barrier function (BF) has been suggested as a cause of reactive follicular wall hyperkeratinization, abnormal desquamation, and follicular plugging or comedo formation.[25,26] Because pilosebaceous units have long canals through which sebum flows, hyperkeratinization of the follicular epithelium easily leads to sebum sequestration, which forms a microenvironment conducive to P acnes proliferation.[26]

Box 1
Summary of the 3 key pathogenic factors in acne

1. Follicular hyperkeratinization
2. Hormonal stimulation of the sebaceous glands
3. Inflammation in response to P acnes

Data from Webster GF. Acne vulgaris and rosacea: evaluation and management. Clin Cornerstone 2001;4(1):15–22.

Two hypotheses suggest that the increased sebum secretion rate (SSR) in AV is associated with the decreased BF and follicular hyperkeratinization that leads to comedo formation. These hypotheses suggest that an increased sebum output dilutes the amount of certain epidermal lipids that are essential components of the SC barrier.[27–29] One hypothesis in particular suggests that patients with AV have lower levels of the essential fatty acid (EFA) linoleic acid compared with healthy skin because of an increased SSR.[30] The hypotheses further propose that relative linoleic/EFA deficiency in the cells of the follicular epithelium[31,32] causes a resultant decrease in follicular epithelial BF,[33] hyperkeratinization of the infundibulum,[26,28,29] and comedo formation.[29] This hypothesis is supported by a measureable inverse relationship between SSR and linoleic content at the skin surface in patients with AV[31,34,35] and more specifically an inverse ratio between SSR and the proportion of linoleate in ceramide 1.[32,34] A second hypothesis, by Melnik and colleagues,[24] suggests that an imbalance of free sterol and cholesterol sulfate secondary to an increased SSR in acne causes follicular retention hyperkeratosis, impaired BF, and comedo formation.

In contrast, other investigators[27,36] have found minimal to no increase in SSR in patients with AV with primarily comedonal lesions or mild AV. In addition, other investigators have found no evidence that SSR affects the composition of ceramide 1 in young adults, aged 15 to 25 years, and also showed no significant difference in the ratio of free sterols to cholesterol sulfate in the SC between patients with AV and control subjects.[24,37] Although it is uncertain whether EFA deficiency and/or altered lipid ratios are caused by an increased SSR in AV, decreased epidermal BF as a pathologic mechanism for follicular plugging has been suggested by other investigators.[27,29,38]

Yamamato and colleagues[27,36] also suggest a comedogenic mechanism involving impaired epidermal BF. In order to prove their hypothesis, Yamamato and colleagues[27,36] determined the SSR, lipid content, and barrier characteristics of the SC in patients with AV. Patients with mild AV had impaired SC permeability BF and decreased sphingolipids (ceramide and free sphingosine) compared with controls with healthy skin. In addition, a correlation was found between decreased sphingolipids and decreased BF in patients with AV. Despite a significant difference in BF between the patients with mild AV and the controls, both groups showed a similar SSR that was significantly lower than that of those patients with moderate AV. This finding suggests that follicular hyperkeratinization and microcomedo formation may still

occur without a high SSR, and that an impaired BF is likely part of the pathophysiology leading to AV lesion formation in patients with mild acne.[38] However, patients with moderate inflammatory AV showed a lower BF and a higher SSR than those with mild AV or a healthy control group.[27,36] Therefore high SSR (and therefore androgens that stimulate a higher SSR) may play more of a pathogenic role in the inflammatory component of moderate to severe AV.

Similar to Yamamoto and colleagues,[27,36] Knutson[38] observed decreased lamellar granules in the infundibulum of comedo-affected follicles compared with the infundibulum of normal follicles. Decreased levels of lamellar granules in the epidermal granular layer lead to reduction in packaging of ceramides and their subsequent release into the SC. Ceramides are an essential component of the intercellular lipid bilayer of the SC, with impaired follicular BF associated with reactive epidermal hyperplasia or hyperkeratosis.[25,27] Knutson[38] and colleagues[26,28] suggested that the decreased ceramide levels, and hence decreased follicular epithelial BF, are related to abnormal follicular hyperkeratinization and comedo formation. The theory of reactive SC hyperkeratinization secondary to impaired epidermal BF has also been suggested in diseases like atopic dermatitis.[17–21] Thus, it is plausible that a similar reaction occurs in the pilosebaceous unit of patients secondary to disturbed follicular BF.[27]

Calcium Gradient

Lee and colleagues[39,40] investigated whether the disruption of the calcium gradient may play a key role in comedogenesis. Calcium is known to play a role in the restoration of BF after skin injury.[39,40] After acute skin barrier impairment, the epidermal calcium gradient is disturbed secondary to loss from the upper epidermis. The loss of calcium from the upper epidermal layers stimulates the self-repair mechanism of lamellar body secretion of lipids into the SC, which promotes epidermal barrier recovery with restoration of the physiologic epidermal calcium gradient.[41] To evaluate the SC intercellular lipids and calcium gradient in the presence of comedonal lesions, Choi and colleagues[28] applied oleic acid on the inner surface of the ears of white rabbits to induce comedo formation, obtained representative specimens, and performed a calcium ion–capture cytochemical procedure with electron microscopy. Incomplete lipid bilayer structures, prominent dilatation of lacunar domains, and the loss of follicular epidermal calcium gradient were identified in the experimentally induced comedos. It was concluded that calcium gradient disruption may play a role in comedo formation in AV pathogenesis.[28]

Subclinical Inflammation

More recent information on the pathophysiology of AV has shown that perifollicular subclinical inflammation is present either before or concurrently with microcomedo formation, suggesting that inflammation may play a role in the development of both comedonal and inflammatory AV lesions.[42,43] The presence of postinflammatory hyperpigmentation after the resolution of comedonal lesions in darker skin types clinically supports the presence of subclinical perifollicular inflammation during the comedonal stage of AV. In addition, initiation of subclinical innate inflammation has been reported to be an initiating event, with increased infiltration of lymphocytes and macrophages with relative absence of neutrophils at the early phase of AV lesion formation.[42,43] It has been suggested that stimulation of the innate immune system is a result of increased bacterial, environmental, and chemical insults that penetrate the impaired follicular barrier; however, confirmatory evidence warrants the support of well-designed studies.[9,10]

In the hypotheses discussed earlier, the unifying concept is that impairment of the follicular barrier plays a contributory role in AV pathophysiology, including during early lesion formation. Whether it is from calcium gradient alteration, SC lipid impairment, or both, follicular barrier dysfunction seems to play a role in both comedonal and inflammatory lesion formation. Perhaps similar to AD, in which impaired epidermal BF is often multifactorial,[44] epidermal barrier dysfunctions involving the pilosebaceous unit wall are significant. Further experimentation is needed.

Androgens

Androgenic hormones play a role in AV pathophysiology because androgens stimulate sebaceous gland proliferation and increased sebum secretion.[45,46] The increased levels of sebum promote an excellent environment for P acnes to proliferate and colonize and, also as discussed earlier, may play a role in comedogenesis.[46] In addition, women with hormonal imbalance (ie, increased androgens) have been known to have significant acneiform eruptions, and therapies designed to decrease androgens are effective for some patients with AV.[45,47] Presence of androgens is associated with emergence of AV; however, most adults with AV have no measurable hormonal imbalance and normal SSRs have been detected in mild acne.[48]

Propionibacterium acnes

P acnes is a commensal bacterium present within in the pilosebaceous unit, with up to 10^7 viable organisms isolated from a single sebaceous unit.[49–51] P acnes predominately exists in the sequestered, lipid-rich, anaerobic environment of the pilosebaceous unit; this bacterium metabolizes sebaceous triglycerides into fatty acids and glycerol[32,49–52] and consumes the glycerol, leaving behind free fatty acids that may serve to promote perifollicular inflammation. The role of P acnes in comedogenesis remains controversial; however, some strains/subtypes of P acnes have been associated with induction of certain proinflammatory pathways.[23,27,38] The observation that abnormal keratinization and comedogenesis can occur in the absence of P acnes does not exclude the possibility that this organism may contribute to microcomedo formation and AV lesion development.

Biofilms

Intrafollicular P acnes microorganisms are capable of encasing themselves in a capsule of extracellular polysaccharide, which they secrete after adherence to the follicular surface, forming what is called a biofilm.[53] Biofilms are composed of populations or communities of bacteria that adhere to environmental surfaces, such as the pilosebaceous unit lining. The extracellular matrix usually comprises most of the biofilm mass and is composed of polysaccharides, water, extracellular DNA, and excreted cellular products.[53] The matrix of the biofilm provides a protective barrier that impedes the penetration of antibiotics. The P acnes biofilm model may provide at least a partial explanation as to why antibiotics are often used over a duration of months in treating AV, whereas much shorter courses are used for standard bacterial infections. However, once antibiotic therapy is stopped, recolonization of P acnes occurs. In addition, it has been shown that there is no correlation between the severity of AV and the levels of P acnes.[53]

The inherent immunologic response of the host and the strains/subtypes of P acnes may explain differences in the severity of inflammation in AV.[54] P acnes instigates inflammatory acne via its interaction with humoral factors, cell mediated immunity, and complement, its secretion of neutrophil and monocyte chemotactic factors, and inducing lysosome enzyme release.[22,54] However, other sources suggest that it is the activation of the innate immune system that initially promotes and influences many of the pathogenic factors in AV.[42,43] **Fig. 1** lists some of the known

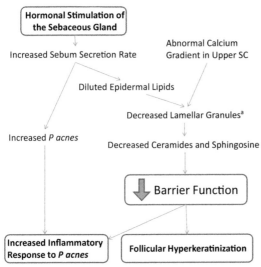

Fig. 1. Summary of the potential role of BF impairment in the 3 key factors of acne pathogenesis. [a] Decreased lamellar granules and decreased ceramide levels may result from causes other than increased SSR. (*Data from* Refs.[22–54])

inflammatory factors that play a role in AV inflammation and pathogenesis.

Although the pathophysiology of AV is still unclear in many ways, the roles of impaired epidermal BF, stimulation of inflammatory cascades, and *P acnes* proliferation are clearer. Therefore it is important to have a cleansing and moisturizing formulation that first and foremost does not contribute to the impairment of BF, inflammation, and growth of *P acnes*.

TOPICAL ACNE PRESCRIPTION THERAPIES AND THE SKIN BARRIER

Topical retinoids and BP are two of the major recognized approaches in AV therapy.[55,56] Despite their proven effectiveness in treating AV, cutaneous irritation associated with their use occurs in many cases, especially with certain formulations, or when adjunctive measures are not used to reduce the risk of local tolerability reactions. The magnitude of cutaneous irritation does vary among patients and with different chemical compounds and/or vehicles.

Topical Retinoids

Topical retinoids are associated with an irritant skin reaction, referred to as retinoid dermatitis, which correlates at least partially with their mechanism of action (MOA).[55,57] In the skin, retinoids stimulate epidermal proliferation and differentiation, which leads to a thickened lower epidermis (or epidermal hyperplasia) with an upper epidermis

(SC) that has greater dyscohesion.[55] The thinning of the SC results clinically in a smoother skin surface, which is associated with altered BF and increased TEWL, especially during the initial few weeks of use.[57] These retinoid-induced changes to the epidermis and the SC account for the scaling, peeling, erythema, dry appearance, and subjective symptoms of skin irritation that are frequently observed in the first few days and weeks of retinoid therapy.[58] The occurrence of cutaneous side effects within the first few weeks of topical retinoid use is thought to be one of the main reasons for nonadherence and treatment failure by patients with AV.[16,59]

Benzoyl Peroxide

BP is one of the most common topical antiacne agents present in many prescription and OTC products.[60] Formulations containing BP include lotions, gels, creams, soaps, and washes, in varying concentrations from 2% to 10% (weight/volume).[60] BP has been shown to have bactericidal properties for *P acnes*,[61] with clinical studies showing that BP improves both inflammatory and comedonal AV lesions.[62] The antimicrobial MOA of BP is secondary to direct oxidative effects on the bacterium; however, this same activity relates to many of the side effects associated with topical use of BP. BP induces peroxidation of SC lipids, which alters SC lipid composition. resulting in impairment of the epidermal barrier.[56,63] Repeated applications of BP can result in SC lipid peroxidation and decreased BF with a significant increase in TEWL.[56,63] The extent of measurable SC lipid peroxidation positively correlates with impairment of SC BF.[63] Another reason for decreased BF with BP use may be damage to SC proteins. It has been shown that BP oxidizes SC proteins, such as keratins 1 and 10, in addition to oxidizing lipids of the SC.[64] Most of these altered SC proteins play a role in the adverse effects on BF.[56]

Given that patients with AV may have inherently impaired epidermal BF and/or barrier dysfunctions related to topically applied agents, properly selected adjunctive skin care mitigates barrier impairment and reduces inflammation. It is for this reason that adjunctive skin care has gained increased recognition as an integral component of AV management. Skin care products that have been properly designed and have been shown to support BF have the potential to ameliorate some of the cutaneous side effects of topical agents used to treat AV (ie, BP, topical retinoids). Reducing adverse side effects associated with AV therapy may foster better patient adherence and achieve better treatment outcomes.

Some of the different types of cleansers available in the marketplace, their potential benefits and detriments, and the clinical evidence that supports the use of well-designed gentle cleansers in AV are reviewed later.

CLEANSER BASICS FOR PATIENTS WITH ACNE

There are 4 general categories of skin cleansing agents: (1) soaps, (2) synthetic detergent (syndet) bars and liquid syndet cleansers, (3) combar antimicrobials, and (4) lipid-free lotion cleansers.

Soaps

True soap is created through a process called saponification, which is the chemical reaction that occurs when a fat, such as tallow (beef fat), and an alkali, such as lye, are combined to create a long chain fatty acid alkali salt. The typical pH of a true soap is 9 to 10.[10] The advantage of cleansing with a true soap is highly effective removal of skin sebum and debris; the disadvantage is removal of, and/or damage to, SC intercellular lipids and proteins. Impaired BF caused by modification of physiologic lipids and proteins induces SC barrier dysfunction, as shown by an increase in TEWL, SC desiccation, and increased penetration of topically applied substances, therefore increasing skin sensitivity and irritation.[10] Interaction of soaps with proteins of the SC also causes a temporary swelling of the corneocytes, which has been suggested as a factor that contributes to follicular plugging and the formation of comedones.[65]

True soap has been shown to increase skin pH,[10,58,66,67] decrease permeability BF,[58,67] alter the bacterial flora,[12,58] dehydrate skin,[58,67] cause erythema and subjective irritation,[10] and cause follicular plugging.[8] Therefore, true soap is not an ideal product to use for cleansing of normal or diseased skin.

Synthetic Detergent Cleansers

Syndet bars are synthetic detergent-based cleansers that contain less than 10% soap and typically have a more neutral/acidic pH (5.5–7), similar to the pH of normal skin.[10,68] Syndet bars in general are designed to provide effective skin cleaning with minimal stripping of the skin's essential lipids and proteins, ultimately making these types of cleansing bars less irritating and drying than traditional soap bars.[68]

In a study by Korting and colleagues,[12] 10 healthy individuals washed their foreheads and forearms twice per day for 8 weeks with either a true soap (Lux soap) or a syndet cleanser (Sebamed Flussig). During the first 4 weeks of the study, half of the individuals washed with the true soap and the other half washed with the syndet cleanser. During the second 4 weeks of the study period, the subjects switched to the other cleanser in a crossover design. Measurements of pH and bacterial flora assessments were obtained every seventh day in both treatment periods. The pH values for the true soap were increased on both the forearm and forehead whether the true soap was used during the first 4-week study period or the second. In contrast, using the syndet cleanser either maintained or decreased skin pH during both study periods. Comparing all the data, the pH values proved to be higher on average when using true soap, by 0.3 pH units ($P<.01$). Bacterial flora assessments showed that the quantification of propionibacteria species was markedly higher when soap was used on both the forehead ($P = .02$) and forearm ($P = .01$). On the forehead there was a clear correlation between bacterial counts and skin pH both with propionibacteria ($P<.001$) and staphylococci ($P<.001$); however, on the forearm, only the former proved true ($P<.05$). The data here are in agreement with other studies, which have shown that repeated use of alkaline soaps increases skin pH[67] and diminishes the ability of the skin to physiologically maintain the normal flora.[66]

There are 2 important conclusions to be drawn from this study by Korting and colleagues.[12] First, that alkaline soap/true soap are best avoided by patients with AV because of the adverse effects of an increased skin pH. Second, when testing products for use in AV, the location of the skin tested may be important because slightly different results were seen with different anatomic locations in this experiment.[12] This second conclusion is supported by other studies that have reported major differences in skin characteristics and behavior patterns based on anatomic location.[69]

Combars

Combars are antibacterial soap bars that contain a combination of true soap surfactants (or syndet bar surfactants) with an added antibacterial agent. Although the antibacterial agents in combars are can reduce harmful bacteria, they may also reduce the normal cutaneous flora, and can cause an increase in skin dryness and irritation.[70] Antiseptic/antibacterial OTC washes such as combars are not generally recommended as adjunctive treatment of AV because most antibacterial ingredients in combars are active primarily against surface gram-positive aerobic bacteria, and washes do not penetrate the follicle enough to achieve a significant and predictable reduction in *P acnes*.[65] In addition, the overuse of these agents has been associated with gram-negative folliculitis.[65,71]

Lipid-free Cleansers

Lipid-free cleansers are the mildest of all the skin cleansers currently on the market because they clean without soap formation[70]; have a neutral to acidic pH; are designed to leave behind a thin moisturizing film on the skin; and generally do not contain dyes, fragrances, or sensitizing preservatives.[58,70]

Syndets and lipid-free cleansers have proved to be beneficial in other skin diseases that are prone to irritation and inflammation, such as atopic dermatitis[9,11] and rosacea,[9,11,67] and therefore are likely to provide the same benefits to patients with AV, especially in the initial treatment phase when the skin is adapting to topical medications. However, within the category of lipid-free cleansers and syndet bars, there are several other properties of these cleansers that determine their mildness. These properties include the type of surfactant used in the cleanser, the extent of the surfactant interactions with skin proteins and lipids, the pH of the cleanser, and the extent of skin hydration or dehydration caused by cleansing.[58,72,73] Therefore, it is important when evaluating these types of cleansers in patients with AV to have clinical evidence supporting their mildness and adjunctive benefits in patients with AV, both alone and concomitantly with AV therapies.

CLINICAL STUDIES EVALUATING THE BENEFITS OF USING MILD CLEANSERS IN ACNE

The following studies investigated the potential benefits of mild cleansers either alone or as an adjuvant treatment in acne therapy.

Bikowski,[58] in his review of the use of cleansers in various skin disorders, including acne, reported a study by Jackson and colleagues[74] that evaluated 3 different cleansing regimens in patients with acne: soap, BP facial cleanser, and an emollient cleanser (brand and manufacturer not reported). All patients used a BP lotion in addition to a cleanser during the study period. Although it was not reported whether the skin was subjectively or objectively assessed in Bikowski's[58] review, it was reported that using the emollient cleanser with the BP lotion resulted in significantly fewer open comedones and inflammatory papules than the soap or BP cleanser with the BP lotion.[74] The improvement seen with the emollient cleanser compared with the BP cleanser and soap may be explained by BP and soap interacting with the skin

barrier and therefore contributing to the pathogenesis of follicular hyperkeratinization and comedo formation or inflammation, as discussed earlier.

Draelos[75] reported a study that evaluated the use of a daily facial cleanser (Cetaphil Daily facial cleanser, Galderma) on the skin of 30 subjects 12 to 50 years old with stable mild facial acne. Stable mild facial acne was defined as less than half the face presenting with many comedones, papules, and pustules. It was hypothesized that the daily facial cleanser would effectively cleanse the skin of patients with acne without compromising the skin barrier or resulting in an overcompensation of sebum.[75] Subjects in the study were instructed to apply a daily facial cleanser twice per day to the whole face for 2 weeks while using no other acne treatments. No other products were allowed during this study period and there was no control in this experiment. Assessments included an evaluation of skin BF, skin sebum level, product tolerability, product performance and likeability, and regimen compliance. Skin BF was assessed with objective measurements with TEWL and corneometry. Sebum level, tolerability assessments, and disease severity were objectively assessed by the investigator at baseline and weeks 1 and 2 using a rating scale of either 0 to 6 or 0 to 4. Lesion counts were also recorded in order to evaluate the product's efficacy. Subjective evaluation of the cleanser's overall rating, ease of use, and perceived efficacy was graded on a scale of 1 to 10.

After using the daily facial cleanser for 2 weeks there was a slightly increased TEWL, although this increase was not significant. Corneometry showed a significant reduction in skin hydration over the course of the study ($P<.001$); however, there was no significant change in sebum level per the investigators assessment and no reported incidences of irritation or intolerability over the course of the study. Investigator lesion counts and assessment of acne severity showed the noncomedogenic/nonacnegenic nature of the cleanser formulation. The mean number of blackheads (open comedones) was 5 at baseline, 2.3 at the end of week 1 ($P = .024$), and 0.1 at the end of the study ($P = .008$). The mean number of total acne lesions was 25 at baseline and 20 at the end of both weeks 1 and 2 ($P = .001$). Five subjects (17%) had a severity score of clear or almost clear at the end of the 2-week study.[63] In the subjective satisfaction survey 17 subjects (57%) rated their satisfaction as 8 or better. Twenty subjects (67%) rated their likeliness of future use at 8 or better, 30 subjects (100%) gave the cleanser a score of 10 for ease of use, and 14 subjects (47%) gave a rating of 8 or better for perceived efficacy. The regimen compliance rate for the study was 99.4%.[75]

The collected data from this study imply that the daily facial cleanser does not significantly affect BF or sebum levels adversely, it is tolerable and does not irritate the skin, and it does not worsen (and may improve) lesion counts and acne severity in patients with mild facial acne. Although there is no doubt that this cleanser is tolerable as a solo therapy in patients with mild acne, the question remains whether this product would be consistently tolerable in a patient who is on additional acne therapy, such as BP or retinoids. Given the lipid-free nature of the daily facial cleanser, it is likely to be tolerable in these patients; however, further experimentation is needed, especially because the TEWL measurements trended upward and skin hydration significantly decreased with use of the daily facial cleanser. These findings may become more of a clinical issue in patients whose barriers are compromised secondary to other medications. It is this authors opinion that the TEWL upward trend or subclinical change in BF may be secondary to the anionic surfactant sodium lauryl sulfate (SLS) in this cleanser's formulation.[75]

Subramanyan[9] reported 2 separate studies involving the evaluation of cleansers in patients with AV. The first study compared the effects of cleansing with a mild syndet bar (Dove sensitive skin bar, Unilever) with true soap in a randomized double-blind study. The study included 50 patients with moderate acne using topical BP-erythromycin gel (Benzamycin) or BP-erythromycin plus adapalene 0.1% gel (Differin) to treat their acne conditions. The patients were instructed to use either a true soap bar or mild syndet bar to cleanse their faces for a 4-week period. The subject's skin was assessed subjectively by the patient and objectively by the investigator for erythema, peeling, dryness, burning, stinging, itching, and tightness, each using a 4-point scale. An overall subjective assessment of acne severity was also collected using a 6-point scale.

The results of the objective assessments at baseline and week 4 showed signs of irritation, especially peeling and dryness, while using the true soap during the 4-week period. Meanwhile, no significant changes in irritation measures were seen for those patients using the syndet bar.

The subjects' assessments for both irritation and acne severity (9 total features) also clearly show that the mild syndet cleanser is more effective in significantly reducing several negative characteristics, such as itching, acne, and oiliness.[9]

In the second randomized double-blind study by Subramayan,[9] 25 patients with acne were recruited and instructed to use a mild cleansing lotion (product name and manufacturer not reported) to cleanse their faces for 4 weeks while continuing to use their acne medications (antibiotics, tretinoin, and/or BP) as normal. It was not mentioned how many times per day the subjects were instructed to cleanse. The subjects' skin conditions were objectively assessed by the dermatologist with regard to acne lesion counts, erythema, and dryness at baseline and at the conclusion of the 4-week study. The results indicate significant decreases in mean scores of key acne-related attributes such as closed comedones and inflammatory papules and pustules with the use of the mild cleansing lotion as well as major improvements in signs of irritation, such as erythema and dryness.[9]

The data in these studies by Jackson and colleagues,[74] Draelos,[75] and Subramanyan[9] show the tolerability and benefit of using mild cleansers rather than true soap in acne. The main benefits of gentle cleansers in acne seem to be an improvement in acne as well as a decrease in the signs and symptoms of irritation.

FREQUENCY OF CLEANSING IN ACNE

As discussed earlier, patients often believe the more the better when it comes to cleansing and their acne, and at one time physicians made similar recommendations.[5,6] The turning point for this common myth concerning cleansing and acne and the resulting the widespread recommendation to avoid overwashing in acne may have been a 1980 study conducted by Swinger and colleagues,[74] which was designed to test whether dryness contributed to acne development. This study showed that moisturizing the skin and avoiding cleansing altogether was more effective at clearing comedones and inflammatory acne lesions than purposely drying the skin with cleansing.[76] Not cleansing at all is generally not recommended by physicians in patients with acne, so the question becomes: how many times per day should patients with acne cleanse?

Most popular acne treatment regimens recommend routinely washing the face twice per day with a mild cleanser. However, even the common recommendation to wash the face twice daily with a mild cleanser has little published scientific evaluation to support its practice.[1]

To clarify the relationship between face washing and AV, a single-blinded, randomized controlled trial on the effect of frequency of face washing on AV was conducted in men with mild to moderate acne.[1] Twenty-seven subjects washed their faces twice daily for 2 weeks with a standard mild facial cleanser (Neutrogena Fresh Foaming Cleanser Neutrogena Corporation, Los Angeles, CA) before being randomized to 1 of 3 study arms, in which face washing was done 1, 2, or 4 times a day for 6 weeks. In contrast with the study by Swinger and colleagues,[76] which showed the less cleansing the better, this study showed a significant worsening of acne in the group that washed their faces once per day and significant improvements in both open comedones and total inflammatory lesions in patients who washed their faces 2 times and 4 times per day. In addition, there was no significant difference in the results seen from those who washed twice per day to those who washed 4 times per day. This study concluded that washing the face more than twice per day does not significantly improve acne[1] and, because of the benefits of convenience and compliance, the twice-per-day recommendation should stand.[1] However, the importance of cleansing in acne is more likely related to the selection of the cleanser than the frequency of washing.

Despite these study results it is the author's opinion that the cleansing regimen should be reduced to twice a day because of the known effects of repeated water exposure to the skin.[66] Excessive use of water alone may disturb the SC, causing dehydration, irritation, changes in skin pH, and alteration of the skin's normal flora.[65,66] Also, cleansing in the morning removes the residue from retinoids and other photoreactive products that are often used at night, whereas cleansing at night removes sunscreen and other cosmetic skin products that may interfere with the absorption of, or inactivate, nighttime acne medications.

DISCUSSION/SUMMARY

This article reviews the pathogenesis of acne, presents the effects of benzoyl peroxide (BPO) and topical retinoids on the skin, and summarizes the available clinical studies investigating the use of gentle cleansers in acne so that clinicians may more thoroughly understand whether gentle cleansers benefit the skin in acne when used with or without acne treatments (Table 1).

Impaired BF may be instrumental in the pathogenesis of AV because decreased BF, whatever the origin, leads to follicular hyperkeratinization, follicular plugging, and comedo formation.[22,25,27] Inflammation, whether the origin is *P acnes* or free fatty acids, is an important component of AV as well.[21] Although excellent progress has been made in the development of effective topical and oral acne therapies to target certain aspects of acne pathogenesis, such as follicular plugging, increased SSR, and *P acnes* proliferation, acne therapies often further aggravate BF and cause further irritation and inflammation in the skin.[55,56]

Table 1
Summary of studies evaluating the benefit of using gentle cleansers in acne

Study	Product Studied	Study Findings
Jackson et al,[74] 1989	• Soap • BPO facial cleanser • Emollient cleanser (brand and manufacturer unknown)	An emollient cleanser with the BPO lotion resulted in significantly fewer open comedones and inflammatory papules than the soap or BPO cleanser with the BPO lotion
Draelos,[75] 2006	• Daily facial cleanser (Cetaphil, Galderma)	The daily facial cleanser does not significantly affect BF or sebum levels adversely, it is tolerable and does not irritate the skin, and does not worsen; it may improve lesion counts and acne severity in patients with mild facial acne
Subramanyan,[9] 2004	• Mild syndet bar (Dove sensitive skin bar, Unilever) • True soap	Objective and subjective assessments show syndet cleanser has significant benefits compared with true soap, such as irritation, dryness, itching, acne, and oiliness
Subramayan,[9] 2004	• Mild cleansing lotion (brand and manufacturer unknown)	The results indicate significant decreases in mean scores of key acne-related attributes, such as closed comedones and inflammatory papules and pustules with use of the mild cleansing lotion as well as major improvements in signs of irritation, such as erythema and dryness

Cleansing is an important aspect of skin care for patients with acne because cleansers have the ability to remove unwanted dirt, oil, and bacteria from skin in addition to preparing skin to absorb topically applied medications by removing dead surface cells.[9] The potential to reduce the level of oil and microbes on skin is of particular relevance to patients with acne. However, it is debatable whether cleansers have the ability to affect oil production and microbial proliferation in the pilosebaceous unit where acne pathogenesis occurs.[65] In addition, cleansers that are designed to strip the skin of oils and kill microbes may further impair BF, contributing to the irritation and inflammation of the skin, altering the pH and normal flora of the skin, and therefore contributing to comedo and acne formation.[27,29,38]

The goals of cleansing in patients with acne are to:

1. Gently cleanse the skin and prepare it for the absorption of topical therapies
2. Avoid skin irritation and dehydration
3. Minimize or reverse the damage to the skin barrier that is seen with many acne therapies
4. Not contribute to the skin comedogenesis or acnegenesis
5. Maintain skin pH
6. Reduce the proliferation and inflammation associated with *P acnes*

The goals of cleansing in acne are summarized in **Box 2**.

Lipid-free and syndet cleansers are designed to meet most if not all of the goals discussed earlier for gentle cleansing in acne. However, as discussed previously, there are several other factors that contribute to a cleanser's mildness within the subtype of lipid-free and syndet cleansers. These properties include the type of surfactant used in the cleanser, the extent of the surfactant's interaction with skin proteins and lipids, the pH of the cleanser, and the extent of skin hydration or dehydration caused by cleansing.[58,72,73] Therefore it is important when evaluating these types of cleansers in patients with acne to have clinical evidence supporting their mildness and benefits, both alone and in addition to acne therapies.

Studies presented here by Jackson and colleagues,[74] Draelos,[75] and Subramanian[9] show that syndet and lipid-free cleansers can improve acne lesion count or acne severity, do not contribute to oiliness of skin, are clinically tolerable and easy to use, and can minimize the irritation seen with other acne therapies such as retinoids and BPO. The recommendation to cleanse the face twice daily in patients with acne remains; however, it was also suggested that the frequency with which patients with acne wash may not be as important as the cleanser selection and the properties of those cleansers.[1] In addition, these studies and others show the minimal effect that lipid cleansers have on many skin properties compared with true soap. True soap can increase skin pH,[10,58,66,67] decrease BF,[58,67] alter the bacterial flora,[12,58] dehydrate skin,[58,67] cause erythema and subjective irritation,[10] and cause follicular plugging,[8] therefore it is not an ideal product to use in most skin diseases, including AV.

Skin cleansing is therefore an important adjuvant to any effective acne therapeutic regimen, and physicians managing AV need to make clear patient recommendations regarding the choice of cleansing product and frequency of use, and dispel myths with regard to acne pathogenesis in order to get optimum efficacy of their prescription medications. This article has shown that gentle cleansers can positively affect AV depending on the type of cleanser used and the frequency of wash, and that gentle cleansing with syndet or lipid-free cleansers can improve treatment efficacy or acne severity, skin irritation and inflammation, skin tolerability, and regimen compliance.

These conclusions, although promising, were made from the few published studies concerning gentle cleansing and acne published from the 1980s to the time of writing. It is surprising that, in such a large span of time, there has been so little experimentation in this arena given the importance of patient perceptions in cleansing and acne. Although the results from this article are promising, further experimentation is needed.

Box 2
Summary of the goals of cleansing in acne

The goals of cleansing in patients with acne are:

1. To gently cleanse the skin and prepare it for the absorption of topical therapies
2. To avoid skin irritation and dehydration
3. To minimize or reverse the damage to the skin barrier seen with many acne therapies
4. Not to contribute to skin comedogenesis or acnegenesis
5. To maintain skin pH
6. To reduce the proliferation and inflammation surrounding of *P acnes*

REFERENCES

1. Choi JM, Lew VK, Kimball AB. A single-blinded, randomized, controlled clinical trial evaluating the effect

of face washing on acne vulgaris. Pediatr Dermatol 2006;23(5):421–7.

2. Mallon E, Newton JN, Klassen A, et al. The quality of life in acne: a comparison with general medical conditions using generic questionnaires. Br J Dermatol 1999;140(4):672–6.

3. Johnson ML, Johnson KG, Engel A. Prevalence, morbidity, and cost of dermatologic diseases. J Am Acad Dermatol 1984;11(5 Pt 2):930–6.

4. Goodman G. Cleansing and moisturizing in acne patients. Am J Clin Dermatol 2009;10(Suppl 1):1–6.

5. Tan JK, Vasey K, Fung KY. Beliefs and perceptions of patients with acne. J Am Acad Dermatol 2001; 44(3):439–45.

6. Green J, Sinclair RD. Perceptions of acne vulgaris in final year medical student written examination answers. Australas J Dermatol 2001;42(2):98–101.

7. Burkhart CG. The role of soap in acne. Dermatol Online J 2006;12(4):19.

8. Mills OH, Klingman AM. Acne detergicans. Arch Dermatol 1975;111(1):65–8.

9. Subramanyan K. Role of mild cleansing in the management of patient skin. Dermatol Ther 2004; 17(Suppl 1):26–34.

10. Ananthapadmanabhan KP, Moore DJ, Subramanyan K, et al. Cleansing without compromise: the impact of cleansers on the skin barrier and the technology of mild cleanser. Dermatol Ther 2004;17:16–25.

11. Hawkins SS, Subramanyan K, Liu D, et al. Cleansing, moisturizing, and sun-protection regimens for normal skin, self-perceived sensitive skin, and dermatologist-assessed sensitive skin. Dermatol Ther 2004;17(Suppl 1):63–8.

12. Korting HC, Kober M, Mueller M, et al. Influence of repeated washings with soap and synthetic detergents on pH and resident flora of the skin of forehead and forearm. Results of a cross-over trial in health probationers. Acta Derm Venereol 1987; 67(1):41–7.

13. Baranda L, González-Amaro R, Torres-Alvarez B, et al. Correlation between pH and irritant effect of cleansers marketed for dry skin. Int J Dermatol 2002;41:494–9.

14. Kuehl BL, Fyfe KS, Shear NH. Cutaneous cleansers. Skin Therapy Lett 2003;8:1–4.

15. Barel AO, Lambrecht R, Clarys P, et al. A comparative study of the effects on the skin of a classical bar soap and a syndet cleansing bar in normal use conditions and in the soap chamber test. Skin Res Technol 2001;7:98–104.

16. Koo J. How do you foster medication adherence for better acne vulgaris management? Skinmed 2003; 2(4):229–33.

17. Spoo J, Wigger-Alberti W, Berndt U, et al. Skin cleansers: three test protocols for the assessment of irritancy ranking. Acta Derm Venereol 2002;82:13–7.

18. Nix DH. Factors to consider when selecting skin cleansing products. J Wound Ostomy Continence Nurs 2000;27:260–8.

19. Loden M. The skin barrier and use of moisturizers in atopic dermatitis. Clin Dermatol 2003;21:145–57.

20. Grove GL, Zerweck C, Pierce E. Noninvasive instrumental methods for assessing moisturizers. In: Leyden JJ, Rawlings AV, editors. Skin moisturization. New York: Marcel Dekker; 2002. p. 499–528.

21. Fluhr J, Holleran WM, Berardesca E. Clinical effects of emollients on skin. In: Leyden JJ, Rawlings AV, editors. Skin moisturization. New York: Marcel Dekker; 2002. p. 223–44.

22. Webster GF. Acne vulgaris and rosacea: evaluation and management. Clin Cornerstone 2001;4(1):15–22.

23. Kligman AM. An overview of acne. J Invest Dermatol 1974;62(3):268–87.

24. Melnik B, Kinner T, Plewig G. Influence of oral isotretinoin treatment on the composition of comedonal lipids. Implications for comedogenesis in acne vulgaris. Arch Dermatol Res 1988;280(2):97–102.

25. Harding CR. The stratum corneum: structure and function in health and disease. Dermatol Ther 2004;17(Suppl 1):6–15.

26. Proksch E, Holleran WM, Menon GK, et al. Barrier function regulates epidermal lipid and DNA synthesis. Br J Dermatol 1993;128(5):473–82.

27. Yamamoto A, Takenouchi K, Ito M. Impaired water barrier function in acne vulgaris. Arch Dermatol Res 1995;287(2):214–8.

28. Choi EH, Ahn SK, Lee SH. The changes of stratum corneum interstices and calcium distribution of follicular epithelium of experimentally induced comedones (EIC) by oleic acid. Exp Dermatol 1997;6(1):29–35.

29. Letawe C, Boone M, Piérard GE. Digital image analysis of the effect of topically applied linoleic acid on acne microcomedones. Clin Exp Dermatol 1998; 23(2):56–8.

30. Morello AM, Downing DT, Strauss JS. Octadecadienoic acids in the skin surface lipids of acne patients and normal subjects. J Invest Dermatol 1976;66(5): 319–23.

31. Wertz PW, Miethke MC, Long SA, et al. The composition of the ceramides from human stratum corneum and from comedones. J Invest Dermatol 1985;84(5):410–2.

32. Downing DT, Stewart ME, Wertz PW, et al. Essential fatty acids and acne. J Am Acad Dermatol 1986; 14(2 Pt 1):221–5.

33. Hou SY, Mitra AK, White SH, et al. Membrane structures in normal and essential fatty acid-deficient stratum corneum: characterization by ruthenium tetroxide staining and x-ray diffraction. J Invest Dermatol 1991;96(2):215–23.

34. Stewart ME, Grahek MO, Cambier LS, et al. Dilutional effect of increased sebaceous gland activity

on the proportion of linoleic acid in sebaceous wax esters and in epidermal acylceramides. J Invest Dermatol 1986;87(6):733–6.

35. Perisho K, Wertz PW, Madison KC, et al. Fatty acids of acylceramides from comedones and from the skin surface of acne patients and control subjects. J Invest Dermatol 1988;90(3):350–3.

36. Yamamoto A, Serizawa S, Ito M, et al. Effect of aging on sebaceous gland activity and on the fatty acid composition of wax esters. J Invest Dermatol 1987; 89(5):507–12.

37. Yamamoto A, Serizawa S, Ito M, et al. Stratum corneum lipid abnormalities in atopic dermatitis. Arch Dermatol Res 1991;283(4):219–23.

38. Knutson DD. Ultrastructural observations in acne vulgaris: the normal sebaceous follicle and acne lesions. J Invest Dermatol 1974;62(3):288–307.

39. Lee SH, Elias PM, Proksch E, et al. Calcium and potassium are important regulators of barrier homeostasis in murine epidermis. J Clin Invest 1992; 89(2):530–8.

40. Lee SH, Elias PM, Feingold KR, et al. A role for ions in barrier recovery after acute perturbation. J Invest Dermatol 1994;102(6):976–9.

41. Menon GK, Elias PM, Lee SH, et al. Localization of calcium in murine epidermis following disruption and repair of the permeability barrier. Cell Tissue Res 1992;270(3):503–12.

42. Krishna S, Kim C, Kim J. Innate immunity in the pathogenesis of acne vulgaris. In: Shalita AR, Del Rosso JQ, Webster GF, editors. Acne vulgaris. New York: Informa Healthcare; 2011. p. 12–27.

43. Jeremy AH, Holland DB, Roberts SG, et al. Inflammatory events are involved in acne lesion initiation. J Invest Dermatol 2003;121:20–7.

44. Elias PM, Schmuth M. Abnormal skin barrier in the etiopathogenesis of atopic dermatitis. Curr Allergy Asthma Rep 2009;9(4):265–72.

45. Berger TG, James WD, Odom RB. Andrew's diseases of the skin. Philadelphia: WB Saunders; 2000.

46. Chen WC, Zouboulis CC. Hormones and the pilosebaceous unit. Dermatoendocrinol 2009;1(2):81–6.

47. Arora MK, Seth S, Dayal S. The relationship of lipid profile and menstrual cycle with acne vulgaris. Clin Biochem 2010;43(18):1415–20.

48. Thiboutot D, Gilliland K, Light J, et al. Androgen metabolism in sebaceous glands from subjects with and without acne. Arch Dermatol 1999;135: 1041–5.

49. Marples RR. The microflora of the face and acne lesions. J Invest Dermatol 1974;62(3):326–31.

50. Nishijima S, Kurokawa I, Katoh N, et al. The bacteriology of acne vulgaris and antimicrobial susceptibility of Propionibacterium acnes and Staphylococcus epidermis isolated from acne lesions. J Dermatol 2000;27(5):318–23.

51. Leyden JJ, McGinley KJ, Mills OH, et al. Propionibacterium levels in patients with and without acne vulgaris. J Invest Dermatol 1975;65(4):382–4.

52. Lavker RM, Leyden JJ, McGinley KJ. The relationship between bacteria and the abnormal follicular keratinization in acne vulgaris. J Invest Dermatol 1981;77(3):325–30.

53. Burkhart CN, Burkhart CG. Microbiology's principle of biofilms as a major factor in the pathogenesis of acne vulgaris. Int J Dermatol 2003;42(12):925–7.

54. Burkhart CG, Burkhart CN, Lehmann PF. Acne: a review of immunologic and microbiologic factors. Postgrad Med J 1999;75(884):328–31.

55. Laquieze S, Czernielewski J, Rueda MJ. Beneficial effect of a moisturizing cream as adjunctive treatment to oral isotretinoin or topical tretinoin in the management of acne. J Drugs Dermatol 2006; 5(10):985–90.

56. Weber SU, Thiele JJ, Han N, et al. Topical alpha-tocotrienol supplementation inhibits lipid peroxidation but fails to mitigate increased transepidermal water loss after benzoyl peroxide treatment of human skin. Free Radic Biol Med 2003;34(2):170–6.

57. Leyden J, Grove G, Zerweck C. Facial tolerability of topical retinoid therapy. J Drugs Dermatol 2004;3(6): 641–51.

58. Bikowski JB. The use of cleansers as therapeutic concomitants in various dermatologic disorders. Cutis 2001;68(5):12–9.

59. Katsambas AD. Why and when the treatment of acne fails. What to do. Dermatology 1998;196(1): 158–61.

60. Ives TJ. Benzoyl peroxide. Am Pharm 1992;NS32(8): 33–8.

61. Leyden JJ, McGinley K, Mills OH, et al. Topical antibiotics and topical antimicrobial agents in acne therapy. Acta Derm Venereol Suppl (Stockh) 1980;(Suppl 89):75–82.

62. Cove JH, Cunliffe WJ, Holland KT. Acne vulgaris: is the bacterial population size significant? Br J Dermatol 1980;102(3):277–80.

63. Man MQ M, Feingold KR, Thornfeldt CR, et al. Optimization of physiological lipid mixtures for barrier repair. J Invest Dermatol 1996;106(5):1096–101.

64. Thiele JJ, Hsieh SN, Briviba K, et al. Protein oxidation in human stratum corneum: susceptibility of keratins to oxidation in vitro and presence of a keratin oxidation gradient in vivo. J Invest Dermatol 1999; 113(3):335–9.

65. Solomon BA, Shalita AR. Effects of detergents on acne. Clin Dermatol 1996;14(1):95–9.

66. Levin J, Maibach H. Human skin buffering capacity: an overview. Skin Res Technol 2008;14(2):121–6.

67. Levin J, Miller R. A guide to the ingredients and potential benefits of over-the-counter cleansers and moisturizers for rosacea patients. J Clin Aesthet Dermatol 2011;4(8):31–49.

68. Draelos ZD. Skin care for the sensitive skin and rosacea patient: the biofilm and new cleansing technology. J Cosmet Dermatol 2006;19(8):520–2.

69. Tagami H. Location-related differences in structure and function of the stratum corneum with special emphasis on those of the facial skin. Int J Cosmet Sci 2008;30(6):413–34.

70. Draelos ZD. Concepts in skin care maintenance. Cutis 2005;76(6 Suppl):19–25.

71. Leyden JJ, Marples RR, Mills OH Jr, et al. Gram-negative folliculitis–a complication of antibiotic therapy in acne vulgaris. Br J Dermatol 1973;88(6): 533–8.

72. Draelos ZD. Facial hygiene and comprehensive management of rosacea. Cuits 2004;73:183–7.

73. Draelos ZD. Cosmetics in acne and rosacea. Semin Cutan Med Surg 2001;20:209–14.

74. Jackson EM, Pack SM, Possick PA, et al. The effect of cleansing regimens on the success of acne therapy using 10% Benzoyl Peroxide lotion. Presented at the meeting of the AAD. Boston, MA, June 26–29 1986.

75. Draelos ZD. The effect of a daily facial cleanser for normal to oily skin on the skin barrier of subjects with acne. Cutis 2006;78(1 Suppl):34–40.

76. Swinyer LJ, Swinyer TA, Britt MR. Topical agents alone in acne. A blind assessment study. JAMA 1980;243(16):1640–3.

Top Ten List of Clinical Pearls in the Treatment of Acne Vulgaris

Alison M. Layton, MB ChB, FRCP (UK)

KEYWORDS

- Acne vulgaris • Topical retinoids • Maintenance therapy • Isotretinoin • Bacterial resistance
- Benzoyl peroxide • Spironolactone • Acne scarring

KEY POINTS

- Target inflammation early in acne management to avoid scarring.
- Consider antibiotic prescribing policies when using antibiotics in the management of acne.
- Identify and treat macrocomedones before commencing oral isotretinoin.
- Isotretinoin absorption depends on fatty food intake.
- Spironolactone may provide an alternative to combined oral contraceptives in female patients who require an antiandrogen therapy.

INTRODUCTION

Acne represents the most common inflammatory dermatosis seen worldwide and is the leading reason for seeing a dermatologist.[1] The disease commonly has a prolonged course, with acute or insidious relapse or recurrence over time and associated social and psychological affects that negatively impact on quality of life.[2] Clinical presentation varies and includes open or closed comedones, papules, pustules, or nodules extending over the face and/or trunk. Discomfort may be a significant manifestation of the inflammatory lesions. Seborrhoea is usually present, although the degree may vary. The combined impact of acne frequently results in psychosocial morbidity. Successful treatment correlates with improvement of psychological factors in many. This article provides a top 10 list of clinical pearls to aid the successful management of acne.

ACNE DURATION AND INFLAMMATION CORRELATE TO THE DEGREE OF SCARRING

There is now clear evidence that acne scarring is more likely to occur if treatment is delayed.[3,4] Recent work presented at the American Academy of Dermatology demonstrated the importance of inflammation in the development of scarring. Both the degree and the duration of clinical inflammation influence resultant scarring.[5]

This emphasizes the need to establish how long the acne has been present when first assessing a patient and to then implement treatment targeting inflammation early in the course of the disease to reduce the likelihood of scarring.

Table 1 outlines an evidence-based algorithm that summarizes treatment options for managing acne. Once under control it is important to consider maintenance therapy with a topical retinoid +/- benzoyl peroxide (BPO). Topical retinoids are the treatment of choice for maintenance

Department of Dermatology, Harrogate and District NHS Foundation Trust, Lancaster Park Road, Harrogate, North Yorkshire HG2 7SX, UK
E-mail address: alison.layton@hdft.nhs.uk

Dermatol Clin 34 (2016) 147–157
http://dx.doi.org/10.1016/j.det.2015.11.008
0733-8635/16/$ – see front matter © 2016 Elsevier Inc. All rights reserved.

Table 1
Algorithm for improving outcomes in acne

	Mild		Moderate		Severe
	Comedonal	Papular/Pustular	Papular/Pustular	Nodular[b]	Nodular/Conglobate
First choice	Topical retinoid	Topical retinoid + topical antimicrobial	Oral antibiotic + topical retinoid ± BPO	Oral antibiotic + topical retinoid ± BPO	Oral isotretinoin[c]
Alternatives[a]	Alt. topical retinoid or Azelaic acid[d] or Salicylic acid	Alt. topical antimicrobial + alt. topical retinoid or Azelaic acid[d]	Alt. oral antibiotic + alt. topical retinoid ± BPO	Oral isotretinoin or Alt. oral antibiotic + alt. topical retinoid ± BPO/azelaic[d] acid	High-dose oral antibiotic + topical retinoid + BPO
Alternatives for females	See first choice	See first choice	Oral antiandrogen + topical retinoid/azelaic acid[d] ± topical antimicrobial	Oral antiandrogen + topical retinoid ± oral antibiotic ± alt. antimicrobial	High-dose oral antiandrogen + topical retinoid ± alt. topical antimicrobial
Maintenance therapy	Topical retinoid	Topical retinoid ± BPO	—	—	—

Abbreviations: Alt., alternative; BPO, benzoyl peroxide.
[a] Consider physical removal of comedones.
[b] With small nodules (>0.5–1 cm).
[c] Second course in case of relapse.
[d] There was not consensus on this alternative recommendation; however, in some countries azelaic acid prescribing is appropriate practice.
Adapted from Nast A, Dreno B, Bettoli V, et al. European evidence-based (S3) guidelines for the treatment of acne. J Eur Acad Dermatol Venereol 2010;26(Suppl 1):8; with permission.

therapy because they impact on the microcomedo that represents the precursor of inflammatory and noninflammatory acne lesions.

ANTIBIOTIC RESISTANCE CAN BE ASSOCIATED WITH REDUCED CLINICAL RESPONSE AND DRIVES RESISTANCE IN *PROPIONIBACTERIUM ACNES* AND OTHER COMMENSAL BACTERIA: CONSIDER ANTIBIOTIC PRESCRIBING POLICIES

There has been a steady rise in antibiotic resistance in *Propionibacterium acnes* as a result of topical antibiotic formulations used for acne[6] and a heavy reliance on antibiotics in long-term acne management. Resistance in *P acnes* is significantly more common to erythromycin and clindamycin than to tetracyclines.[7] In the United Kingdom the only community study conducted confirmed that 47% of 649 patients were colonized by erythromycin-resistant propionibacteria and 41% by clindamycin-resistant strains, whereas only 18% were colonized by strains resistant to tetracyclines.[8] Resistance rates in hospital settings globally are much higher.[9]

Once colonized with resistant propionibacteria the resultant effect is most likely to be a reduced response or relapse rather than no response at all. However, studies have clarified that the carriage of antibiotic-resistant strains reduces the efficacy of systemic erythromycin and to a lesser extent oral tetracyclines.[8–10]

In the United States the prevalence of antibiotic resistance to oral macrolides has rendered them far from useful in the management of acne. The situation as a result of topical antibiotics used in acne is less clear, although a reduction in the efficacy of topical erythromycin over time has been demonstrated in a meta-analysis.[11] Although acne is not infectious, antibiotic-resistant *P acnes* are transmissible between subjects by person-to-person transfer of pre-existing resistant strains. This can result in an untreated person being colonized with resistant strains potentially making them less susceptible to antibiotic treatment.[6]

Antibiotics may also impact on pathogens other that *P acnes*. Studies have previously demonstrated profound changes in the resident flora of skin and nonskin sites during antibiotic therapy for acne. Oral antibiotic therapy exposes all body sites with a resident commensal flora to selective pressure. When delivery is topical, selective pressure for the overgrowth of resistant strains and species is largely confined to the skin. Antibiotic-resistant strains of coagulase-negative staphylococci rapidly replace susceptible strains on the skin and in the anterior nares during oral and topical antibiotic therapy for acne.[12]

Increased numbers of coagulase-negative staphylococci resistant to multiple antibiotics have also been found on the skin of untreated contacts of patients with acne managed with sequential antibiotics.[13] Similarly, increased numbers of coliforms, such as *Escherichia coli* resistant to multiple antibiotics, have been found in the gastrointestinal tracts of patients with acne and their relatives during treatment with oral tetracycline.[14] The judicious use of antibiotics is essential when prescribing for acne and antibiotic prescribing policies are now advocated in the management of acne (**Table 2**).

The efficacy of some combined topical therapies rivals that of oral tetracyclines. Prescribing a fixed-dose combination product may also improve adherence and guarantees concomitant use of both drugs. Combination therapy is not usually required for mild acne; BPO or a topical retinoid (tretinoin, isotretinoin, or adapalene) are treatments of choice and are selected according to apparent lesion type, with retinoids being superior in treating comedonal lesions. BPO can be used as a stand-alone treatment for mild papulopustular acne. It is a more potent antibacterial than antibiotics and is highly effective in rapidly reducing propionibacteria whether sensitive or resistant strains are present.[15]

ACUTE FLARE OF ACNE ON COMMENCING ORAL ISOTRETINOIN: BE AWARE OF THE MACROCOMEDONE

The most common reason for an acute acne flare after commencing oral isotretinoin relates to the presence of macrocomedones (**Fig. 1**).[16] Macrocomedones may be subtle particularly in the context of significant inflammation. Examination should be done under suitable lighting with the skin stretched. Once identified isotretinoin should be delayed or commenced at a very low dose until macrocomedones have been treated with light cautery or hyfrecation.[17]

If patients still suffer an acne flare at the start of a course of isotretinoin, an antibiotic can be used in combination with oral isotretinoin (eg, erythromycin, 1 g daily, or trimethoprim, 200 to 300 mg twice daily). Tetracyclines should not be combined with isotretinoin because of a possible increased risk of benign intracranial hypertension.[18,19] If the acne is very inflammatory, then low-dose isotretinoin (0.2–0.4 mg/kg/day) alongside oral steroids (0.5–1.0 mg/kg/day) may be required.

Persistent deep pustules may reflect *Staphylococcus aureus* in approximately 1% of patients.

Table 2
Antibiotic prescribing policies for acne: limit antibiotic usage to preserve antibiotic sensitivity

Strategy to Avoid Propionibacterial Resistance Emerging	Comments
Avoid inappropriate use of topical and systemic antibiotics	Use oral antibiotics for 3 months in the first instance and only continue if clinical improvement continues
If extending the duration of oral antibiotics use combination therapy	Combine with an agent that reduces the likelihood of promoting antibiotic propionibacterial resistance (eg, benzoyl peroxide)
If repeated courses of antibiotics are required and the initial clinical response was favorable, reuse the same drug	This avoids multiple resistant strains emerging
Avoid prescribing different oral and topical antibiotics concomitantly	This avoids multiple resistant strains emerging
Consider using topical retinoids and nonantibiotic antimicrobials wherever possible	These do not promote resistant isolates and when used with antibiotics may achieve more rapid efficacy so reduce the duration of the antibiotic course
Topical BPO is fully active against sensitive and resistant strains of *P acnes* and able to eradicate resistant isolates	BPO can be used for 7 days between antibiotic courses; short contact BPO seems to be more efficacious for clearing *P acnes* on the trunk than BPO washes
Remember to check medical adherence	Poor adherence to antibiotic therapies promotes resistance

A bacterial swab should be performed and antistaphylococcal therapy prescribed alongside the oral isotretinoin.

ISOTRETINOIN ABSORPTION IS FOOD DEPENDENT. AN EMPTY STOMACH MAY REDUCE ABSORPTION LEADING TO A SIGNIFICANT REDUCTION IN BLOOD LEVELS: ENSURE PATIENTS KNOW HOW TO TAKE ISOTRETINOIN BECAUSE THIS MAY IMPACT ON SAFETY, EFFICACY, AND DURATION OF THERAPY

The half-life of isotretinoin is 22 hours. Early studies with oral isotretinoin found that it was 1.5 to 2 times more bioavailable with food ingested 1 hour before, concomitantly with, or 1 hour after dosing than when given during a complete fast. Absorption is markedly affected by the presence of fat and pharmacokinetic studies show that if no food is ingested with isotretinoin the fasting plasma levels of isotretinoin after intake of standard oral formulations can be up to 60% lower than levels obtained in the fed state.[20] This may have a significant impact on efficacy and safety. Isotretinoin capsules should therefore be taken with fatty food at the same time of day. The dose can then be adjusted according to clinical response and presence or absence of side effects.[21]

Posttherapy relapse is said to be minimized by treatment courses that amount to a total of least 120 to 150 mg/kg, with greater than 150 mg/kg not providing a better therapeutic response for acne.[22–24] The duration of therapy varies according to the dose administered over the course of the treatment period. The range is usually 16 to 30 weeks, and the mean between 16 and 20 weeks, with patients receiving 0.5 mg/kg/day requiring a longer course of therapy to achieve previously recommended cumulative dosing and desired clinical results. Early studies aimed at deriving a cumulative dose for maximum benefit

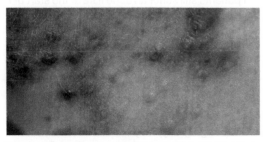

Fig. 1. Flare of acne post start of isotretinoin in context of macrocomedones.

and reduced relapse rate confirmed an effect of dose and duration of therapy but not a pharmacokinetic reason to support the concept of accumulation of drug or a cumulative dose effect.[25] Recent publications suggest that the dose should be tailored to the tolerability of the drug and the clinical response and have demonstrated that the cumulative doses previously recommended may not be necessary in all patients or be achieved if patients are not taking the drug appropriately. There may be significant differences in the absorption of the drug determined by diet in different individuals. Novel formulations less dependent on fatty food for absorption have been developed and are undergoing efficacy and safety assessments, but when prescribing a generic form the importance of ingesting oral isotretinoin with food to maximize bioavailability should be emphasized and the duration of therapy should be adjusted to give at least 90% clearance of acne based on initial clinical acne grade scoring techniques followed by 4 to 8 weeks of consolidation.

CONSIDER HOW TO MANAGE ADVERSE EFFECTS AND INTERACTIONS OF TOPICAL AGENTS TO OPTIMIZE EFFICACY: AVOID IRRITATION, COSMETIC ISSUES CAUSED BY INTERACTIONS AS WITH DAPSONE AND BENZOYL PEROXIDE OR SULFACETAMIDE OR INSTABILITY WHEN USING TRETINOIN AND BENZOYL PEROXIDE

The most common side effect of topical acne products is a primary irritant dermatitis, which often subsides with time and is managed by reducing frequency of application, using emollients and if severe, short-term application of a type I potency topical corticosteroid.[26,27]

Other interactions to be aware of when combining topical agents include a yellow/orange discoloration of the skin and hair when topical dapsone or sulfacetamide are combined with BPO applied within a short time frame.[28] The color easily wipes away and does not stain skin; however, it is advisable to use these agents at different ends of the day and to ensure the BPO is completely removed before applying other agents. The exact mechanism involved in this reaction remains unclear. Another recognized reaction is the oxidation, degradation, and inactivation of certain formulations of tretinoin by BPO. This reaction is accelerated when these formulations are exposed to light.[29] It is important to be aware of any possible cross-reactions because these may impact on efficacy and adherence.

EVIDENCE TO SUPPORT HIGH-DOSE DOXYCYCLINE PLUS A FIXED COMBINATION PRODUCT AS AN ALTERNATIVE TO ORAL ISOTRETINOIN IN SEVERE NODULAR ACNE

Oral isotretinoin is the treatment of choice for severe inflammatory acne with nodules. The many potential side effects of isotretinoin, increasing regulatory controls, and public anxiety can result in patients not wishing to embark on treatment with systemic isotretinoin. To date there have been a paucity of studies available to support alternatives to isotretinoin in the treatment of severe acne.

A recent multicenter randomized, parallel group controlled, investigator-blinded trial was conducted to comparing the efficacy/safety profile of a fixed-dose combination of topical adapalene 0.1%/BPO 2.5% gel plus doxycycline, 200 mg/d, with vehicle gel plus oral isotretinoin, 0.5 mg/kg/day, for 30 days followed by 1 mg/kg/day in the treatment of severe acne with nodules.[30] Inclusion criteria included patients with severe facial acne (investigator global assessment [IGA] $\geq$4), with five or more nodules and 20 or more inflammatory lesions (papules and pustules). A total of 266 subjects were randomized. Most patients completed the study.

Both treatment regimens were found to be highly efficacious and safe in the treatment of severe nodular acne (**Fig. 2**). The fixed topical combination plus doxycycline arm showed rapid onset of action and greater efficacy in reducing lesions at 2 weeks when compared with oral isotretinoin; however, oral isotretinoin was superior at Week 20.

The retinoid/BPO plus doxycycline combination had superior safety profile, less related serious adverse effects, and fewer related adverse effects requiring treatment during the course of the study. When adverse effects did occur they were of lower severity when compared with those resulting from isotretinoin.

No increase of atrophic acne scars was reported in either group, suggesting a comparable effect on prevention of atrophic acne scars. This was expected in the oral isotretinoin group but not in the combination group and is thought to relate to the more rapid impact of the combination group on inflammation, that is, clinical improvement was noted at 2 weeks and/or could be the positive impact of tetracyclines on matrix metalloproteinases known to be involved in the process of scarring. Patient-reported outcomes reflected the clinical results and confirmed the comparability of the two regimens when considering the efficacy/safety profiles of both treatments. In summary, when a 75% reduction of lesions was

Ada/BPO + Doxycycline

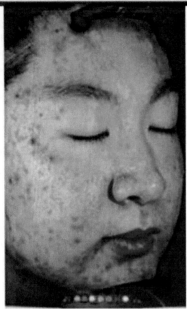 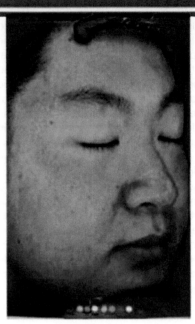

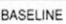

BASELINE   WEEK 20

Fig. 2. High-dose doxycycline for acne; baseline versus Week 20. Ada, adapalene; BPO, benzoyl peroxide.

considered, fixed combination of adapalene/ BPO plus doxycycline (200 mg) demonstrated a comparable benefit/risk to isotretinoin over 20 weeks in the treatment of severe acne with nodules. This combination approach provides an alternative treatment option for nodular acne in those unwilling, unable, or intolerant of isotretinoin.[30]

ANTIHISTAMINES AMELIORATE THE ADVERSE EFFECTS OF ORAL ISOTRETINOIN AND ACT AS AN ADJUVANT IN THE MANAGEMENT OF MODERATE TO SEVERE ACNE

Histamine has a possible role in acne pathogenesis by working as an inflammatory mediator in the immune reaction implicated in acne pathogenesis and has also been shown in vitro to decrease lipogenesis in sebocytes.[31] A recent study investigated the efficacy and safety of combining oral isotretinoin with antihistamine and compared this combination with oral isotretinoin used as monotherapy.

Forty patients with moderate to severe acne were recruited into a randomized controlled comparative study. Twenty received oral isotretinoin alone at a dose of 20 mg daily and the second group received oral isotretinoin at the same dose

with 5 mg desloratadine. Results confirmed that at Week 12 the isotretinoin plus desloratadine group demonstrated a more statistically significant decrease in acne lesion counts, global grading, and measured values of erythema and sebum. In addition acne flare was less frequent and adverse effects of isotretinoin more tolerable in the group taking additional antihistamine. Patient satisfaction was significantly greater in the group receiving both treatments.

These early results provide some evidence that antihistamine has a complementary effect and reduces adverse effects of isotretinoin and as such antihistamine may be used as an adjuvant treatment alongside systemic isotretinoin in moderate to severe acne.[32]

SPIRONOLACTONE AS AN ALTERNATIVE TO COMBINED ORAL CONTRACEPTIVES IN FEMALE PATIENTS WHO REQUIRE AN ANTIANDROGEN THERAPY

An increasing number of postteenage women are seeking treatment advice for their acne. Postadolescent acne fails to respond to conventional therapy in more than 80% of cases and relapse following isotretinoin occurs in up to 30% of cases.[33]

Spironolactone is reported in the literature as an effective treatment of acne. Through the ability to inhibit sebaceous gland activity it reduces sebum excretion by 30% to 75% depending on the dosage used. It is also able to decrease 5α-reductase activity via increased clearance of testosterone secondary to augmented liver hydroxylase activity and increases the level of steroid hormone binding globulin hence reducing the circulating free testosterone. At a local level spironolactone competes with dihydrotestosterone for cutaneous androgen receptors thereby inhibiting testosterone and dihydrotestosterone binding. Many women with late-onset or persistent teenage acne do not exhibit an increase in serum androgens. However, spironolactone has been reported as efficacious in these patients and provides an alternative therapy in this subgroup, particularly those that present with a characteristic clinical pattern of disease manifested as predominance of inflammatory papules concentrated around the lower half of the jawline, chin, and cheeks.

Box 1 summarizes potential clinical indications where oral spironolactone may prove of benefit in women with postteenage acne. Underlying systemic cause of hyperandrogenism should be considered and relevant clinical history and drug history should be taken into account when considering treatment with spironolactone.

Spironolactone is usually prescribed at a dose of 50 to 100 mg daily with meals, but many women with sporadic outbreaks do well with doses of 25 mg daily.[34–37] Although spironolactone is used in this context with clinical success there are a paucity of studies to confirm evidence of its effectiveness because of small sample populations studied and poor trial design.[38] One small study confirmed efficacy and good tolerability in 27 women with severe papular and nodulocystic acne treated with a combination of ethinyl estradiol, 30 μg, and drospirenone, 3 mg, and 100-mg spironolactone suggesting augmented benefit by combining the two agents.[39]

The main side effects are menstrual irregularity, breast tenderness, occasional fluid retention, and rarely melasma. A question mark remains regarding long-term use because of a theoretic increase in breast cancer, which has been shown in animal but not human studies.[40] A measured approach with potential avoidance in those with a personal history of breast cancer and/or a family history in a first-degree relative is advised.[33] Pregnancy should be avoided because of potential abnormalities to the male fetus. Serum electrolytes should be monitored in older women who might have other medical problems because of potential risk of hyperkalemia. It is advisable to avoid the combined use of spironolactone with trimethoprim-sulfamethoxazole because there are reports of both agents leading to hyperkalemia and coadministration with lithium may lead to an increased level of serum lithium and associated toxicity.

LONG-TERM ANTIBIOTICS MAY LEAD TO GRAM-NEGATIVE FOLLICULITIS

Gram-negative folliculitis (**Fig. 3**) can result as a consequence of any long-term topical or oral antibiotic therapy. It results from an overgrowth of gram-negative organisms including *Klebsiella, E coli, Proteus, Serratia,* or *Pseudomonas* organisms.[41] Clinically two forms of gram-negative folliculitis have been described.[42] Type 1 may

---

Box 1
Potential clinical indications for oral spironolactone

Females with clinical signs of hyperandrogenism (eg, hirsutism, increased seborrhoea, androgenic alopecia)

Females with late-onset acne or persistent acne, with or without signs of hyperandrogenism

Females not responding to conventional therapy who do not wish to take oral isotretinoin or cannot take isotretinoin

Females with acne flares that mirror the menstrual cycle

Females who may not be able to take oral contraceptives but require an antiandrogen as part of their acne regimen

Females on oral contraceptives who manifest signs of moderate to severe acne

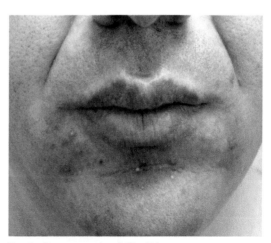

Fig. 3. Gram-negative folliculitis.

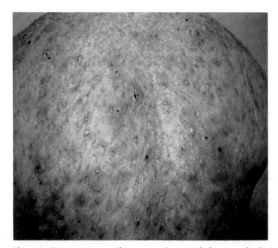

Fig. 4. Severe truncal acne triggered by anabolic steroids.

present with an acute flare of many pustules, predominantly around the nose and chin. Alternatively, type 2 represents an apparent deterioration of ordinary acne characterized by more painful, deep pustules and nodules, some of which may coalesce to form sinus tracts. *Proteus mirabilis* is frequently isolated from this second form. Bacterial swabs should be sampled from the skin and nose of these patients to identify the organism implicated. The current antibiotic should be stopped. Alternative antibiotic treatment options include ampicillin, 250 mg three times per day, or oral trimethoprim, 200 to 300 mg twice a day. However, systemic isotretinoin, 0.5 to 1.0 mg/kg/day, is the treatment of choice because relapse after antibiotic therapy is much more frequent.

Table 3
Top 10 clinical pearls for managing acne

Duration of acne and inflammation correlate with scarring	Early effective treatment aimed at managing inflammation is important
Judicious use of antibiotics is essential to preserve antibiotic sensitivity	High resistance to macrolides has made them much less effective in the management of acne
Acute acne flare postisotretinoin frequently relates to the presence of macrocomedones	Identification with a suitable acne lamp and treatment with cautery or hyfrecation are required before proceeding with oral isotretinoin
Isotretinoin absorption depends on food, especially fatty food; no food may lead to up to a 60% reduction in absorption	Patients should be instructed to take their medication with fatty foods at the same time of day to ensure appropriate absorption
Manage adverse effects of topical agents and recognize interactions to optimize efficacy	Topical agents are frequently irritant; good advice on emollient usage and incremental duration of application can enhance tolerability Be aware of any interactions between topical agents
Fixed-dose combination BPO/adapalene + doxycycline has been shown to be effective in severe nodular acne	An alternative option in severe disease with nodules
Antihistamines provide an effective adjuvant therapy alongside isotretinoin and reduce adverse effects	Increase tolerability and enhanced efficacy achieved
Spironolactone offers an option in women with postadolescent hormonal acne	Selection of spironolactone requires a careful history and appreciation of any underlying medical problems and other medications being taken
Gram-negative folliculitis may result from long-term antibiotic usage	May be mistaken for a flare of acne in the context of long-term antibiotic usage
Beware of anabolic steroids, nutritional, and vitamin supplements as a trigger for acne	Patients do not often consider over-the-counter and nonprescribed products to be medicinal agents

BE AWARE OF ANABOLIC STEROIDS, NUTRITIONAL, AND VITAMIN SUPPLEMENTS AS A TRIGGER FOR ACNE OR ACNEIFORM ERUPTIONS

Abuse of androgenic anabolic steroids, synthetic derivatives of testosterone, and testosterone salts by bodybuilders and others can exacerbate acne vulgaris (Fig. 4) and induce severe forms of acne fulminans or acne conglobata.[43–51] Usage of androgenic anabolic steroids is increasing. The induction of acne is caused at least in part by androgen receptor binding leading to hypertrophy of the sebaceous glands with consequent increased sebum output and a concomitant increase in the population density of P acnes.[52–55] Estimates suggest that 43% of users have some degree of acne as a side effect.[46]

Protein shakes and similar nutritional supplements, which are also widely and easily available, can also induce acne in men and women.[56,57] They consist of whey protein extracts, which often contain bioactive amounts of transforming growth factor, insulinlike growth factor 1 and 2, platelet-derived growth factor, and fibroblast growth factor 1 and 2. In a prospective open study, a pronounced worsening of acne and an increase in acne prevalence was observed among 30 adults who used protein calorie supplements for 2 months.[58] Twenty-two percent of users of nutritional supplements reported acne as a side effect.[59]

Vitamins B_2, B_6, and B_{12}

Exacerbation or new-onset of acne has been described with B_{12} doses of 5 to 10 mg per week. Women are almost exclusively affected and the onset of acne develops within the first 2 weeks after the injection. The acne-inducing dose of B_6 has not been established. Iodine is present in some ampoules of B_{12} and may be the trigger. The eruption is monomorphic consisting of small follicular papule and pustules on the face especially the forehead and chin, upper arms, and upper trunk.[60]

Conventional acne therapies are usually unsuccessful but the acneiform rash settles within 8 to 10 days of withdrawing the vitamin B therapy. Table 3 summarizes the top 10 clinical pearls for acne described in this article.

REFERENCES

1. Stern S. Dermatologists and office-based care of dermatologist disease in the 21st century. J Investig Dermatol Symp Proc 2004;9:126–30.

2. Thiboutot D, Gollnick H, Bettolli V, et al. New insights into the management of acne: an update from the Global Alliance to Improve Outcomes in Acne Group. J Am Acad Dermatol 2009;60:s1–50.

3. Layton AM, Henderson C, Cunliffe WJ. A clinical evaluation of acne scarring and its incidence. Clin Exp Dermatol 1994;19:303–8.

4. Tan JK, Tang J, Fung K, et al. Development and validation of a comprehensive acne severity scale. J Cutan Med Surg 2007;11(6):211–6.

5. Bourdes V, Faure C, Petot L, et al. Natural history of acne lesions and atrophic acne scars within a 6 month study period. Presented at American Academy of Dermatology. San Francisco, March 20–24, 2015.

6. Leyden JJ, Del Rosso JQ, Webster GF. Clinical considerations in the treatment of acne vulgaris and other inflammatory skin disorders: a status report. Dermatol Clin 2009;27:1–15.

7. Coates P, Vyakrnam S, Eady EA, et al. Prevalence of antibiotic-resistant propionibacteria on the skin of acne patients: 10-year surveillance data and snapshot distribution study. Br J Dermatol 2002;146:840–8.

8. Ozolins M, Eady EA, Avery A, et al. Comparison of five antimicrobial regimens for treatment of mild to moderate facial inflammatory acne vulgaris in the community: a randomized controlled trial. Lancet 2004;364:2188–95.

9. Leyden JJ, McGinley KJ, Cavalieri S, et al. Propionibacterium acnes resistance to antibiotics in acne patients. J Am Acad Dermatol 1983;8:41–5.

10. Eady EA, Cove JH, Holland KT, et al. Erythromycin resistant propionibacteria in antibiotic treated acne patients: association with therapeutic failure. Br J Dermatol 1989;121:51–7.

11. Simonart T, Dramaix M. Treatment of acne with topical antibiotics: lessons from clinical studies. Br J Dermatol 2005;153:395–403.

12. Harkaway KS, McGinley KJ, Foglia AN, et al. Antibiotic resistance patterns in coagulase negative staphylococci after treatment with topical erythromycin, benzoyl peroxide and combination therapy. Br J Dermatol 1992;126:586–90.

13. Miller YW, Eady EA, Lacey RW, et al. Sequential antibiotic therapy for acne promotes the carriage of resistant staphylococci on the skin of contacts. J Antimicrob Chemother 1996;38:829–37.

14. Adams SJ, Cunliffe WJ, Cooke EM. Long-term antibiotic therapy for acne vulgaris: effects on the bowel flora of patients and their relatives. J Invest Dermatol 1985;85:35–7.

15. Kircik LH. The role of benzoyl peroxide in the new treatment paradigm for acne. J Drugs Dermatol 2013;12:s73–6.

16. Clark SM, Cunliffe WJ. Acne flare and isotretinoin—incidence and treatment. Br J Dermatol 1995;133(Suppl 45):26.

17. Pepall LM, Cosgrove MP, Cunliffe WJ. Ablation of whiteheads by cautery under topical anesthesia. Br J Dermatol 1991;125:256–9.

18. Griffin JP. A review of the literature on benign intracranial hypertension associated with medication. Adverse Drug React Toxicol Rev 1992;11:41–58.

19. Lee AG. Pseudotumor cerebri after treatment with tetracycline and isotretinoin for acne. Cutis 1995; 55:165–8.

20. Colburn WA, Gibson DM, Wiens RE, et al. Food increases the bioavailability of isotretinoin. J Clin Pharmacol 1983;23:534–8.

21. Del Rosso JQ. Face to face with oral isotretinoin; a closer look at the spectrum of therapeutic outcomes and why some patients need repeated courses. J Clin Aesthet Dermatol 2012;5(11):17–24. QUESTIONS • CHALLENGES • CONTROVERSIES.

22. Strauss JS, Krowchuk DP, Leyden JJ, et al. Guidelines of care for acne vulgaris management. J Am Acad Dermatol 2007;56(4):651–63.

23. Layton AM. The use of isotretinoin in acne. Dermatoendocrinol 2009;1(3):162–9. QUESTIONS • CHALLENGES • CONTROVERSIES 2012;5(11).

24. Cryulnik AA, Viola KV, Gewirtzman AJ, et al. High-dose isotretinoin in acne vulgaris: improved treatment outcomes and quality of life. Int J Dermatol 2012;51:1123–30.

25. Harms M, Masooye I, Radeff B. The relapses of cystic acne after isotretinoin treatment are age-related: a long-term follow up study. Dermatologica 1986;172:148–53.

26. Olsen TE. Therapy of acne. Med Clin North Am 1982;66:851–77.

27. Sykes NL, Webster GF. Acne: a review of optimum treatment. Drugs 1994;48:59–70.

28. Dubina M, Fleisher AB. Interaction of topical sulfacetamide and topical Dapsone with benzoyl peroxide. Arch Dermatol 2009;145(9):1027–9.

29. Martin B, Meunier C, Montels D, et al. Congenital alopecia areata. J Am Acad Dermatol 1998;139(Suppl 52):8–11.

30. Tan J, Humphrey S, Vender R, et al, The POWER Study Group. A treatment for severe nodular acne: a randomised investigator-blinded, controlled, non-inferiority trial comparing fixed-dose Adapalene/BPO plus doxycycline vs oral isotretinoin. Br J Dermatol 2014;171(6):1508–16.

31. Pelle E, McCarthy J, Seltmann H, et al. Identification of histamine receptors and reduction of squalene levels by an antihistamine in sebocytes. J Invest Dermatol 2007;128:1280–5.

32. Lee HE, Chang IK, Lee CD, et al. Effect of antihistamine as an adjuvant treatment of isotretinoin in acne: a randomised, controlled comparative study. J Eur Acad Dermatol Venereol 2014;28:1654–60.

33. Kim G, Del Rosoo JQ. Oral spironolactone in postteenage female patients with acne vulgaris practical considerations for the clinical based on current data and clinical experience. Clin Aesthet 2012;5(31):37–50.

34. Muhlemann MF, Carter GD, Cream JJ, et al. Oral spironolactone: an effective treatment for acne vulgaris in women. Br J Dermatol 1986;115:227–32.

35. Goodfellow A, Alaghband-Zadeh J, Carter C, et al. Oral spironolactone improves acne vulgaris and reduces sebum excretion. Br J Dermatol 1984;111:209–14.

36. Lubbos H, Rose LI. Adverse effects of spironolactone therapy in women with acne. Arch Dermatol 1998;134:1162–3.

37. Thiboutot D. Acne: hormonal concepts and therapy. Clin Dermatol 2004;22:419–28.

38. Farquhar C, Lee O, Toomath R, et al. Spironolactone versus placebo or in combination with steroids for hirsutism and/or acne. Cochrane Database Syst Rev 2003;(4):CD000194.

39. Krunic A, Ciurea A, Scheman A. Efficacy and tolerance of acne treated with both spironolactone and a combined contraceptive containing drospirenone. J Am Acad Dermatol 2008;58:60–2.

40. Loube SD, Quirk RA. Breast cancer associated with administration of spironolactone. Lancet 1975;1:1428–9.

41. Fulton JE, McGinley K, Leyden J. Gram negative folliculitis in acne. Arch Dermatol 1968;98:349–53.

42. Leyden JJ, Marples RR, Mills OH, et al. Gram negative folliculitis—a complication of antibiotic therapy in acne vulgaris. Br J Dermatol 1973;88:533–8.

43. Heydenreich G. Testosterone and anabolic steroids and acne fulminans. Arch Dermatol 1989;125:571–2.

44. Collins P, Cotterill JA. Gymnasium acne. Clin Exp Dermatol 1995;20:509.

45. Evans NA. Gym and tonic: a profile of 100 male steroid users. Br J Sports Med 1997;31:54–8.

46. O'Sullivan AJ, Kennedy MC, Casey JH, et al. Anabolic-androgenic steroids: medical assessment of present, past and potential users. Med J Aust 2000;173:323–7.

47. Eklof AC, Thurelius AM, Garle M, et al. The anti-doping hot-line, a means to capture the abuse of doping agents in the Swedish society and a new service function in clinical pharmacology. Eur J Clin Pharmacol 2003;59:571–7.

48. Walker SL, Parry EJ. Acne induced by 'Sus' and 'Deca'. Clin Exp Dermatol 2006;31:297–8.

49. Melnik B, Jansen T, Grabbe S. Abuse of anabolic-androgenic steroids and bodybuilding acne: an underestimated health problem. J Dtsch Dermatol Ges 2007;5:110–7.

50. Voelcker V, Sticherling M, Bauerschmitz J. Severe ulcerated 'bodybuilding acne' caused by anabolic steroid use and exacerbated by isotretinoin. Int Wound J 2010;7:199–201.

51. Razavi Z, Moeini B, Shafiei Y, et al. Prevalence of anabolic steroid use and associated factors among body-builders in Hamadan, west province of Iran. J Res Health Sci 2014;14:163–6.

52. Kiraly CL, Alen M, Rahkila P, et al. Effect of androgenic and anabolic steroids on the sebaceous gland in power athletes. Acta Derm Venereol 1987; 67:36–40.

53. Kiraly CL, Collan Y, Alen M. Effect of testosterone and anabolic steroids on the size of sebaceous glands in power athletes. Am J Dermatopathol 1987;9:515–9.

54. Kiraly CL, Alen M, Korvola J, et al. The effect of testosterone and anabolic steroids on the skin surface lipids and the population of *Propionibacterium acnes* in young postpubertal men. Acta Derm Venereol 1988;68:21–6.

55. Scott MJ, Scott AM. Effects of anabolic-androgenic steroids on the pilosebaceous unit. Cutis 1992;50:113–6.

56. Silverberg NB. Whey protein precipitating moderate to severe acne flares in 5 teenaged athletes. Cutis 2012;90:70–2.

57. Simonart T. Acne and whey protein supplementation among bodybuilders. Dermatology 2012;225:256–8.

58. Pontes Tde C, Fernandes Filho GM, Trindade Ade S, et al. Incidence of acne vulgaris in young adult users of protein-calorie supplements in the city of Joao Pessoa - PB. An Bras Dermatol 2013;88:907–12.

59. Da Silva WV, de Andrade Gomes Silva MI, Tavares Toscano L, et al. Supplementation prevalence and adverse effects in physical exercise practitioners. Nutr Hosp 2014;29:158–65.

60. Dupre A, Alberel N, Bonafe JL, et al. Vitamin B-12 induced acnes. Cutis 1979;24(2):210–1.

Use of Oral Contraceptives for Management of Acne Vulgaris
Practical Considerations in Real World Practice

Julie C. Harper, MD

KEYWORDS

• Acne vulgaris • Hormones • Oral contraceptives • Hyperandrogenism

KEY POINTS

• Combination oral contraceptive pills (COCs) are effective at reducing acne in women.
• COCs are useful for women with and without clinical and/or laboratory signs of hyperandrogenism. It is important to do an appropriate hormonal laboratory work-up in women with clinical signs or symptoms of hyperandrogenism to exclude underlying conditions such as late-onset congenital adrenal hyperplasia, polycystic ovary syndrome, and adrenal or ovarian androgen-secreting tumors.
• All COCs are associated with an increased risk of venous thromboembolism compared to the age-matched population.
• Blood pressure measurement should be performed prior to initiating therapy with a COC. Papanicolaou smears and bimanual pelvic examinations are not required to initiate treatment with a COC.
• There are contraindications to COC use including pregnancy, hypertension, migraine headaches, and cigarette smoking in women over the age of 35.

The pathogenesis of acne is complex and multifactorial. Androgen hormones and excess sebum may contribute to the development of acne and are potential targets for treatment. Combination oral contraceptive pills (COC's) are indirectly anti-androgenic and they have been used with success in the treatment of acne.[1] It is important that dermatology providers understand when and how to prescribe these medications safely and effectively.

COMBINATION ORAL CONTRACEPTIVE PILLS

Combination oral contraceptives contain a combination of ethinyl estradiol and a progestin. The ethinyl estradiol dose ranges from 10 µg to 50 µg per day. The progestational agent employed in COCs varies widely from pill to pill. Most of the first- and second-generation progestins (ie, norethindrone, norethindrone acetate, levonorgestrel) are derived from testosterone and may interact with the progesterone receptor, the androgen receptor, the estrogen receptor, the glucocorticoid receptor, and the mineralocorticoid receptor. Although these progestins are successful at preventing pregnancy, they may produce adverse effects related to this nonspecific receptor selectivity.[2] Third-generation progestins, including desogestrel, norgestimate, and gestodene, are also derived from

The Dermatology and Skin Care Center of Birmingham, 2470 Rocky Ridge Road, Birmingham, AL 35243, USA
E-mail address: juharper@yahoo.com

Dermatol Clin 34 (2016) 159–165
http://dx.doi.org/10.1016/j.det.2015.11.005
0733-8635/16/$ – see front matter

testosterone but have been modified to be less androgenic.[3] Fourth-generation progestins, including drospirenone, bind specifically to the progesterone receptor and not to the other steroid receptors, resulting in no androgenic adverse effects.[2] Drospirenone is derived from 17-alpha spironolactone and has antiandrogenic and antimineralocorticoid effects.

The overall androgenic effect of a COC may be influenced by the type and dose of progestin, by the dose of estrogen, and by its overall suppressive effects on the ovary. Although fourth-generation progestins are, by themselves, antiandrogenic, there is evidence that COCs containing first-, second-, third-, and fourth-generation progestins result in a net increase in sex hormone binding globulin (SHBG) and a net decrease in free testosterone.[4]

MECHANISM OF ACTION IN ACNE

The antiandrogenic effects of COCs may be useful in the treatment of acne. COCs decrease production and activity of androgens through several mechanisms. First, COCs suppress the gonadotropins, luteinizing hormone (LH), and follicle-stimulating hormone (FSH). This suppresses ovarian production of androgen and ovulation. Second, ethinyl estradiol increases hepatic synthesis of SHBG. SHBG binds free testosterone (T) and prevents it from binding to the androgen receptor or from being converted to the more potent dihydrotestosterone (DHT). Third, some progestins inhibit 5-alpha reductase, which converts T to DHT.[5]

EFFICACY IN ACNE

There have been numerous studies that evaluate the efficacy of COCs in the treatment of acne. A large Cochrane meta-analysis recently evaluated 31 of these studies. Of 10 trials that included a placebo group, 9 trials showed improvements in acne, and 1 trial had insufficient data to analyze. The progestins included in these placebo-controlled trials included levonorgestrel (LNG), norethindrone acetate (NA), norgestimate (NGM), drospirenone (DRSP), dienogest, and chlormadinone acetate (CMA). Seventeen of the remaining trials compared 2 COCs in the treatment of acne. COCs containing CMA or cyproterone acetate, neither of which are available in the United States, seem to work better for acne than those containing LNG. COCs containing DRSP seem to work better than those containing NGM or nomegestrel acetate. The authors concluded that comparisons between other

COCs were either conflicting or showed no significant difference in acne reduction.[1]

The usefulness of COCs in truncal acne has also been evaluated. DRSP/ethinyl estradiol 20 μg was shown to be superior to placebo for truncal acne in a 24-week study. Noninflammatory, inflammatory, and total lesion counts diminished by 52.1%, 53.2%, and 57.3% with DRSP/ethinyl estradiol 20 μg compared with -9.2%, 18.2%, and 17% with placebo (P=.02, .05, and .02, respectively).[6]

Four COCs are currently US Food and Drug Administration (FDA)-approved for the treatment of acne. They are Ortho Tri-Cyclen (norgestimate 0.180 mg, 0.215 mg, 0.250 mg/ethinyl estradiol 35 μg), Estrostep Fe (norethindrone acetate 1 mg/ethinyl estradiol 20 μg, 30 μg, 35 μg and ferrous fumarate), Yaz (drospirenone 3 mg/ethinyl estradiol 20 μg) and Beyaz (drospirenone 3 mg/ethinyl estradiol 20 μg and levomefolate calcium). It is important to understand the nuances of these FDA indications. All of the COCs FDA-approved for acne are FDA-approved for acne in women who also desire contraception. Balancing the risks of COCs against the risks of pregnancy is quite different from balancing the risks of COCs against the risks of acne.

BENEFITS

COCs offer many noncontraceptive benefits. They normalize the menstrual cycle, reduce anemia, reduce the risk of ectopic pregnancy, reduce pelvic inflammatory disease, and decrease endometrial, ovarian, and colorectal cancer risks.[7] Ovarian cancer risks are decreased by 40% in women 20 to 54 years of age who have taken a COC for even just a few months versus women who have never taken a COC.[8] This protective effect persists long after the COC is discontinued.[9] Endometrial cancer risk is decreased by about 50% in COC users versus never users.[10]

Premenstrual dysphoric disorder symptoms may also be lessened with COCs. In particular, a Cochrane meta-analysis concluded that COCs containing drospirenone 3 mg and ethinyl estradiol 20 μg may help reduce the symptoms of premenstrual dysphoric disorder.[11]

RISKS

COCs are not without risks. They increase the risk of venous thromboembolism (VTE), myocardial infarction, and stroke. They also have an impact on cervical and breast cancer risks. There is ongoing debate about their role in bone mineral density and bone mass accrual.

Cardiovascular Risks

Certainly the risk that has garnered the most attention recently is the risk of VTE. All COC use increases the risk of VTE compared with nonuse, and higher estrogen doses are associated with higher risks. A Cochrane meta-analysis of combined oral contraceptives and venous thrombosis found that all COCs investigated were associated with an increased risk of venous thrombosis. This increased risk was dependent on both the progestin and the dose of ethinyl estradiol. COCs with 30 to 35 μg of ethinyl estradiol and gestodene, desogestrel, cyproterone acetate, and drospirenone were similar and 50% to 80% higher than with levonorgestrel.[12] There have been much conflicting data on this topic, but other studies have concluded that newer-generation progestins, including drospirenone, may be associated with a greater risk of VTE than other progestins.[13] Jick and colleagues[14] reported that the risk of nonfatal VTE associated with COCs containing drospirenone is about twice that of COCs containing levonorgestrel. The FDA conducted its own investigation and also found an increased VTE risk associated with drospirenone as compared with various other progestins.[15] It is important, however, to keep this increased risk in perspective. The overall absolute risk of VTE remains small with all COCs. According to a Committee Opinion from The American College of Obstetricians and Gynecologists, the risk of VTE is increased among COC users to 3 to 9 events per 10,000 woman–years compared with 1 to 5 events per 10,000 woman–years in nonusers who are not pregnant. The risk associated with drospirenone containing COCs may be 10.22 events per 10,000 woman–years. This should be weighed against the risk of VTE during pregnancy (5–20 per 10,000 woman–years) and the postpartum period (40–65 per 10,000 woman-years).[16] Again, the risk of VTE associated with a COC may be well worth it when the COC is being used to prevent pregnancy. Consider these risks thoughtfully when prescribing a COC for acne in a woman who does not need contraception.

There are several high-risk factors that may increase the risk of VTE associated with COC use. These include smoking and age 35 years or older, less than 21 days post-partum or 21 to 42 days postpartum with other risk factors, major surgery with prolonged immobilization, history of deep vein thrombosis or pulmonary embolism, hereditary thrombophilia, inflammatory bowel disease with active or extensive disease, surgery, immobilization, corticosteroid use, vitamin deficiencies or fluid depletion, and systemic lupus erythematosus with positive or unknown antiphospholipid antibodies.[16]

The World Health Organization (WHO) states that current or prior use of a COC is not associated with increased risk for myocardial infarction in healthy nonsmokers.[17] Cigarette smoking and COC use may increase the relative risk of myocardial infarction by up to 30-fold. COCs are contraindicated in women 35 years or older who smoke. Hypertension is another independent risk factor for myocardial infarction in COC users.[7]

Both ischemic and hemorrhagic stroke may be increased in COC users. Cigarette smoking, hypertension, and a history of migraine increase the risk of ischemic stroke, as do ethinyl estradiol doses of 50 μg or more. In COC users over the age of 35, smoking and hypertension also increase the risks of hemorrhagic stroke.[7]

Cancer Risks

A large meta-analysis of 54 studies analyzed the role of COCs in the development of breast cancer. The relative risk (RR) of having breast cancer diagnosed in current users was 1.24 (95% confidence interval [CI] 1.15–1.33). The cancers diagnosed in women who had used COCs were less advanced clinically than those diagnosed in never users. There was no significant increased risk of breast cancer diagnosed 10 or more years after stopping the COC.[18] A 2013 review of oral contraceptive use and the risk of breast cancer also concluded that the risk of breast cancer was slightly elevated for women who ever used a COC versus never users. In contradistinction to the risk of VTE, this slight increase risk may translate to a more substantial absolute risk, because the baseline incidence of breast cancer is high.[19]

Cervical cancer risks may be increased in COC users. Results from 24 pooled studies analyzing this potential risk concluded that the RR of cervical cancer in current COC users increases with increasing duration of use. After 5 years of COC use, the risk doubles. This increase in risk vanishes after 10 years without COC use.[20]

Liver cancer risks are increased with COC use, while colorectal cancer risks are decreased.[7,19]

Bone Risks

Low estrogen (20 μg ethinyl estradiol or less) COCs may result in estrogen levels too low for young adolescents to develop optimal bone mass. This appears to be most important when starting a low estrogen COC within 3 years from menarche and using the COC for more than 2 years continuously. There is strong evidence that COCs containing 30 µg of ethinyl estradiol or more do not have a negative impact on bone accrual during adolescence.[21]

CONTRAINDICATIONS

COC use is contraindicated in some women (**Box 1**).[22] Absolute contraindications to their use include pregnancy, history of thromboembolic or heart disease, liver disease, and active smoking in women 35 years of age or older. Relative contraindications also include hypertension, diabetes, migraine, breastfeeding, and current breast or liver cancer.[22] As a dermatologist prescribing COCs for acne, I do not prescribe these medications to anyone with either an absolute or relative contraindication. Individuals with a relative contraindication to the use of a COC may still benefit from a COC, but I refer these patients to a specialist in obstetrics/gynecology.

WHEN TO USE

Androgen hormones play an important role in the pathophysiology of acne. COCs, with their antiandrogen effects, may be beneficial to any

woman with acne who does not have a known contraindication to their use. COCs may be used first line in women who also desire contraception or when added to an existing acne regimen where results are unsatisfactory. COCs may be prescribed for acne in women who do not need contraception, but the risk/benefit ratio should be considered and discussed with the patient prior to their use. Remember that the risks of COCs are less than the risks associated with pregnancy. When assessing the risks of COCs versus the risks of acne, consider the severity of acne and its resistance to other available treatments.

Although most women with acne have normal circulating androgen levels, some will have hyperandrogenism. The presence of resistant acne, hirsutism, alopecia, and oligomenorrhea or amenorrhea can signal hyperandrogenism and should prompt a laboratory evaluation (**Table 1**).[23] This includes free and total testosterone, sex hormone binding globulin (SHBG), and dehydroepiandrosterone sulfate (DHEA-S). Elevated 17-hydroxyprogesterone can confirm a diagnosis of C-21 hydroxylase deficiency. An elevated LH to FSH ratio may also help to confirm a diagnosis of polycystic ovary syndrome (PCOS). In women who are also anovulatory, TSH and prolactin should also be checked. These laboratory tests should be obtained during the menstrual flow when possible, and any hormonal therapy should be discontinued at least 1 month prior to the evaluation.[24] PCOS is the most common cause of hyperandrogenism in women, and COCs are the first-line pharmacologic therapy for this condition in women who are not trying to become pregnant.[25] Other sources of excess androgen can be adrenal or ovarian androgen-secreting tumors and late-onset congenital adrenal hyperplasia (nonclassical C21-hydroxylase deficiency).[23] These conditions should be excluded in women with hyperandrogenism prior to treatment with COCs.

HOW TO USE

COCs may be useful in any woman with acne in the absence of any known contraindications. It is important to review these contraindications with all potential COC users to eliminate unnecessary risks.[22] Aside from a typical dermatology examination, the only additional physical examination recommendation is to measure and record blood pressure prior to prescribing a COC.[26] A bimanual pelvic examination and Papanicolaou smear are not mandatory prior to treating with a COC.[22,25] As mentioned earlier, signs of hyperandrogenism should prompt an appropriate work-up.

Box 1
Contraindications to the use of combination oral contraceptive pills

Pregnancy

Breastfeeding less than 6 months postpartum

History of venous thromboembolic disease

Smoking and greater than 35 years of age

History of migraine and greater than 35 years of age (or <35 years of age but with focal neurologic symptoms)

Uncontrolled hypertension

Diabetes and greater than 35 years of age (or <35 years of age but with end-organ damage)

History of stroke

History of ischemic heart disease

Current or personal history of breast cancer

Hypercholesterolemia

Viral hepatitis

Cirrhosis

Liver tumor (benign or malignant)

Major surgery with prolonged immobilization

Table 1
Laboratory screening evaluation for hyperandrogenism

Total Testosterone	Marker of overall androgen production A portion of total testosterone is bound and biologically inactive Total testosterone measures all testosterone and is not the ideal measurement for biologically active testosterone Testosterone levels fluctuate during the day and should be measured in the morning	Mild elevations may be seen in PCOS and CAH Striking elevations (>200 ng/dL) suggest tumorous production (ovary or adrenal)
Free Testosterone	This represents the unbound, biologically active testosterone; it is the preferred measurement but there is some variability in both the way testosterone in measured or calculated	Mild elevations may be seen in PCOS and CAH Striking elevations (>200 ng/dL) suggest tumorous production (ovary or adrenal)
SHBG	Binds testosterone SHBG is primarily used to calculate free testosterone	Levels may be decreased in PCOS
DHEA-S	Marker of adrenal androgen production	Elevations may be seen in PCOS and CAH Striking elevations (>700 μg/dL) suggest adrenal tumor production
LH (FSH)	Gonadotropins that promote both ovarian androgen production and ovulation LH and FSH are suppressed by combination oral contraceptive pills	Can be used as a confirmatory laboratory measurement LH:FSH >2 may be seen in PCOS
17-hydroxyprogesterone	Adrenal cortisol pathway byproduct that is, proximal to the C-21 hydroxylase enzyme	Can be use as a confirmatory laboratory measurement if DHEA-S is elevated 17-hydroxyprogesterone is elevated in non-classical C-21 hydroxylase deficiency (late-onset CAH); it will also increase further with an ACTH stimulation test in late-onset CAH

The first four rows represent recommended initial screening laboratory tests. LH/FSH and 17-hydroxyprogesterone may be evaluated to further characterize the source of excess androgen. The initial screening examination should be performed during the morning hours and, when possible, during menses. All hormonal medications should be discontinued for at least 1 month prior to performing a hormonal laboratory work-up.

COCs may be used first line in women with acne who also desire contraception.

Even then, they may be used in combination with more traditional medications including topical retinoids and/or antibiotics. COCs may take 3 cycles of use to show an effect in acne lesion count reductions.[27-30] Combining COCs with other acne medications with a quicker onset of action may be of benefit in some cases based on my experience. Antibiotics typically prescribed for acne have not been shown to lessen the effectiveness of a COC's ability to prevent pregnancy.[31]

Rifampin and griseofulvin are antimicrobials that can lessen the effectiveness of COCs.[32]

The Sunday start or the quick start methods are 2 simple ways to initiate treatment with a COC. The Sunday start method requires that the woman wait until her next menses and then take her first pill on the subsequent Sunday, even if she is still bleeding. Starting the COC during menses ensures that the woman is not pregnant when the COC is initiated. Alternatively, the quick start method allows the first pill to be taken immediately after a negative pregnancy test.[33] The package insert of COCs contains valuable information regarding missed pills. I instruct patients to familiarize themselves with these recommendations. Even if the COC is not being used for contraception, it is important to take the pill as prescribed to minimize unwanted adverse effects, like unscheduled bleeding.

I generally ask acne patients to return to clinic for an initial follow-up at 8 weeks. Although COCs may not have had sufficient time to show significant results in acne, this visit still allows me to address any adverse effects or concerns that the patient may be experiencing. At the 16-week follow-up, I expect to see improvement in acne. By the end of 6 to 9 cycles of the COC, I will begin tapering off other acne medications when applicable. Acne in many of my patients is well-controlled with a COC as mono-therapy. It is important to encourage acne patients treated with a COC to have a well woman examination, including a pelvic examination, breast examination, and Papanicolaou smear when appropriate. It is recommended that the first screening for cervical cancer occur within 3 years of the initiation of sexual intercourse or by the age of 21 years, whichever occurs first.[25]

ADVERSE EFFECTS

Adverse effects of COC use may include nausea, breast tenderness, and unscheduled or breakthrough bleeding. These adverse effects may be experienced early in treatment, and women should be encouraged to continue taking the COC. To minimize unscheduled or breakthrough bleeding, remind COC users to take pills at roughly the same time every day as scheduled and to avoid missing pills.[34]

Potential weight gain is of particular importance to potential COC users. Interestingly, a Cochrane meta-analysis has analyzed the data regarding COCs and their effects on weight. Three placebo-controlled, randomized trials showed no evidence supporting a causal association between COCs or a combination skin patch and weight gain. Most comparative studies failed to show a difference in weight gain, and discontinuation of the drug based on weight did not differ between groups.[35]

REFERENCES

1. Arowojolu AO, Gallo MF, Lopez LM, et al. Combined oral contraceptive pills for treatment of acne. Cochrane Database Syst Rev 2012;(7):CD004425.
2. Sitruk-Ware R. Pharmacology of different progestogens: the special case of drospirenone. Climacteric 2005;8(Suppl 3):4–12.
3. Davtyan C. Four generations of progestins in oral contraceptives. Proceedings of UCLA Healthcare 2012;16:1–3.
4. Koulianos GT. Treatment of acne with oral contraceptives: criteria for pill selection. Cutis 2000;66: 281–6.
5. Rabe T, Kowland A, Ortmann J, et al. Inhibition of skin 5 alpha reductase by oral contraceptive progestins in vitro. Gynecol Endocrinol 2000;14:223–30.
6. Palli MB, Reyes-Habito CM, Lima XT, et al. A single-center, randomized double-blind, parallel-group study to examine the safety and efficacy of 3mg drospirenone/0.02mg ethinyl estradiol compared with placebo in the treatment of moderate truncal acne vulgaris. J Drugs Dermatol 2013;12(6):633–7.
7. Burkman R, Schlesselman JJ, Zieman M. Safety concerns and health benefits associated with oral contraception. Am J Obstet Gynecol 2004; 190:S5–22.
8. The reduction in risk of ovarian cancer associated with oral-contraceptive use. The Cancer and Steroid Hormone Study of the Centers for Disease Control and the National Institute of Child Health and Human Development. N Engl J Med 1987;316:650–5.
9. Maguire K, Westhoff C. The state of hormonal contraception today: established and emerging noncontraceptive health benefits. Am J Obstet Gynecol 2011;205(4 Suppl):S4–8.
10. Weiss NS, Sayvetz TA. Incidence of endometrial cancer in relation to the use of oral contraceptives. N Engl J Med 1980;302:551–4.
11. Lopez LM, Kaptein AA, Helmerhorst FM. Oral contraceptives containing drospirenone for premenstrual syndrome. Cochrane Database Syst Rev 2012;(2):CD006586.
12. deBastos M, Stegeman BH, Rosendaal FR, et al. Combined oral contraceptives: venous thrombosis. Cochrane Database Syst Rev 2014;(3):CD010813.
13. Raymond EG, Burke AE, Espey E. Combined hormonal contraceptives and venous thromboembolism: putting the risks into perspective. Obstet Gynecol 2012;119(5):1039–44.
14. Jick SS, Hernandez RK. Risk of non-fatal venous thromboembolism in women using oral contraceptives containing drospirenone compared with women using oral contraceptives containing levonorgestrel: a case-control study using United States claims data. BMJ 2011;342:d2151.
15. FDA Office of Surveillance and Epidemiology. Combined hormonal contraceptives and the risk of cardiovascular disease endpoints. 2011. Available at: http://www.fda.gov/downloads/Drugs/Drug. Accessed March 01, 2015.
16. Committee on Gynecologic Practice. ACOG Committee Opinion No. 540. Risk of venous thromboembolism among users of drospirenone-containing oral contraceptive pills. Obstet Gynecol 2012;120:1239–42.

17. WHO. Cardiovascular disease and steroid hormone contraception: report of a WHO Scientific Group. Geneva (Switzerland): WHO Scientific Group on Cardiovascular Disease and Steroid Hormone Contraception; 1998. WHO Technical Report No. 877.

18. Collaborative Group on Hormonal Factors in Breast Cancer. Breast cancer and hormonal contraceptives: collaborative reanalysis of individual data on 53,297 women with breast cancer and 100,239 women without breast cancer from 54 epidemiological studies. Lancet 1996;347: 1713–27.

19. Gierisch JM, Coeytaux RR, Peragallo Urrutia R, et al. Oral contraceptive use and trisk of breast, cervical, colorectal, and endometrial cancers: a systematic review. Cancer Epidemiol Biomarkers Prev 2013; 22(11):1931–43.

20. International Collaboration of Epidemiological Studies of Cervical Cancer, Appleby P, Beral V, et al. Cervical cancer and hormonal contraceptives: collaborative reanalysis of individual data for 16,573 women with cervical cancer and 35,509 women without cervical cancer from 24 epidemiological studies. Lancet 2007;370:1609–21.

21. Agostino H, DiMeglio G. Low-dose oral contraceptives in adolescents: how low can you go? J Pediatr Adolesc Gynecol 2010;23:195–201.

22. Frangos JE, Alavian CN, Kimball AB. Acne and oral contraceptives: update on women's health screening guidelines. J Am Acad Dermatol 2008; 58:781–6.

23. Somani N, Harrison S, Bergfeld W. The clinical evaluation of hirsutism. Dermatol Ther 2008;21:376–91.

24. Harper JC. Evaluating hyperandrogenism: a challenge in acne management. J Drugs Dermatol 2008;7(6):527–30.

25. Buzney E, Sheu J, Buzney C, et al. Polycystic ovary syndrome: a review for dermatologists Part II Treatment. J Am Acad Dermatol 2014;71:859.e1–15.

26. Stewart FH, Harper CC, Ellertson CE, et al. Clinical breast and pelvic examination requirements for hormonal contraception. JAMA 2001;285(17):2232–9.

27. Koltun W, Maloney JM, Marr J, et al. Treatment of moderate acne vulgaris unsing a combined oral contraceptive containing ethinylestradiol 20µg plus drospirenone 3 mg administered in a 24/4 regimen: a pooled analysis. Eur J Obstet Gynecol Reprod Biol 2011;155:171–5.

28. Maloney JM, Dietze P, Watson D, et al. A randomized controlled trial of a low-dose combined oral contraceptive containing 3 mg drospirenone plus 20µg ethinyl estradiol in the treatment of acne vulgaris: lesion counts, investigator ratings and subject self-assessment. J Drugs Dermatol 2009;8(9):837–44.

29. Lucky AW, Koltun W, Thiboutot D, et al. A combined oral contraceptive containing 3mg drospirenone/ 20µg ethinyl estradiol in the treatment of acne vulgaris: a randomized, double-blind, placebo-controlled study evaluating lesion counts and participant self-assessment. Cutis 2008;82:143–50.

30. vanVloten WA, vanHaselen CW, van Zuuren EJ, et al. The effect of 2 combined oral contraceptives containing either drospirenone or cyproterone acetate on acne and seborrhea. Cutis 2002;69(4S):2–15.

31. London BM, Lookingbill DP. Frequency of pregnancy in acne patients taking oral antibiotics and oral contraceptives. Arch Dermatol 1994;130:392–3.

32. Weisberg E. Interactions between oral contraceptives and antifungals/antibacterials; is contraceptive failure the result? Clin Pharmacokinet 1999;36(5): 309–13.

33. Brahmi D, Curtis KM. When can a woman start combination hormonal contraceptives (CHCs)?: a systematic review. Contraception 2013;87(5):524–38.

34. Tyler KH, Zirwas MJ. Contraception and the dermatologist. J Am Acad Dermatol 2013;68:1022–9.

35. Gallo MF, Lopez LM, Grimes DA, et al. Combination contraceptives: effects on weight. Cochrane Database Syst Rev 2008;(4):CD003987.

The Clinical Relevance of Antibiotic Resistance

Thirteen Principles That Every Dermatologist Needs to Consider When Prescribing Antibiotic Therapy

James Q. Del Rosso, DO[a],*, Joshua A. Zeichner, MD[b]

KEYWORDS

• Antibiotic resistance • Antibiotic therapy • MRSA • Propionibacterium acnes

KEY POINTS

• The use of oral or topical antibiotics induces selection pressure, which favors the persistence of bacteria that are less sensitive to the antibiotic administered, and sometimes to other similar antibiotics that are susceptible to cross-resistance mechanisms.
• The emergent antibiotic-resistant bacteria may include commensal flora and transient pathogenic flora, including *Staphylococcus aureus* and *Streptococcus pyogenes*.
• In management of acne vulgaris, use of oral and topical antibiotics as monotherapy is not recommended. Concomitant use of benzoyl peroxide (BP) can reduce the emergence of antibiotic-resistant *Propionibacterium acnes* strains. This occurs only at anatomic sires where BP is applied and does not reduce emergence of resistant bacteria exposed to antibiotic in the mouth, gastrointestinal, and genitourinary tracts.
• Overall reduction in prescribing of specific antibiotics and classes in a geographic community correlates directly with a decrease in the prevalence of resistant bacterial strains.
• Subantimicrobial dosing of doxycycline has been shown to exhibit anti-inflammatory properties, which seem to at least partially explain efficacy in papulopustular rosacea. Efficacy and safety in patients with papulopustular rosacea and AV, and lack of antibiotic selection pressure are supported by a large body of scientific evidence.

MAJOR PREMISE #1: DERMATOLOGISTS ARE THE MOST COMMON PRESCRIBERS OF ANTIBIOTIC THERAPY IN THE UNITED STATES

Principle #1: Antibiotic therapy is most commonly used by dermatologists to treat noninfectious inflammatory dermatoses, such as acne vulgaris (AV) and rosacea.

Principle #2: Durations of therapy with antibiotic use for many inflammatory dermatoses are often prolonged over several weeks to months.

Principle #3: Antibiotic resistance is a consistent and unavoidable adverse effect associated with systemic and topical antibiotic use. The emergence of serious infections caused by bacteria that are highly resistant to many previously effective antibiotics necessitates that all clinicians consider when an antibiotic truly needs to be used and to prescribe judiciously.

Topical and oral antibiotics are commonly used by dermatologists in clinical practice, primarily

[a] Dermatology, Touro University Nevada, 874 American Pacific Drive, Henderson, NV 89014, USA;
[b] Department of Dermatology, Icahn School of Medicine at Mount Sinai, 5 East 98 Street, 5th Floor, New York, NY 10029, USA
* Corresponding author.
E-mail address: jqdelrosso@yahoo.com

Dermatol Clin 34 (2016) 167–173
http://dx.doi.org/10.1016/j.det.2015.12.003
0733-8635/16/$ – see front matter © 2016 Elsevier Inc. All rights reserved.

because of the overall track record of favorable efficacy and safety with the most commonly used agents (ie, tetracyclines, macrolides).[1] Among categories of physicians in the United States including primary care and specialty areas, dermatologists prescribe more oral antibiotics per practitioner than any other physician group based on data collected by the US Centers for Disease Control and Prevention (CDC).[2] The types of antibiotics that are commonly prescribed also differ among dermatologists compared with other physician types, with approximately three-fourths of all oral antibiotic prescriptions in the United States being written for a tetracycline agent (usually doxycycline or minocycline).[1–4] The higher frequency of oral antibiotic prescribing and the differences in the types of antibiotics used by dermatologists compared with other physicians are because dermatologists commonly use tetracycline agents to treat common inflammatory skin diseases, especially AV and rosacea.[1–6] Importantly, when oral antibiotics are used to treat AV and rosacea, they are frequently administered for prolonged durations of therapy over several weeks to months, compared with short courses used to treat common infections, such urinary tract infections, upper respiratory tract infections, otitis media, and uncomplicated skin/soft tissue infections.[1–4] The use of oral antibiotic therapy to treat AV, especially the tetracycline agents doxycycline and minocycline, remains part of published guidelines on the management of AV, and is also included among recommended therapies for treatment of papulopustular rosacea.[5–10] Because antibiotic resistance is an unavoidable sequelae of their systemic or topical administration, it is important that all clinicians take this into account when considering use of and selecting antibiotic therapy.[2–4]

Over the past decade, increased attention has been given to the problems associated with antibiotic resistance, especially with the emergence of methicillin-resistant *Staphylococcus aureus*, macrolide-resistant staphylococci and streptococci, and hospital-based pathogens, such as enterococci and *Clostridium difficile*, which have acquired antibiotic resistance patterns that create major therapeutic challenges.[11–13] In addition, the marked decrease over the past few decades in development of antibiotics, especially new drug classes, has been a major impetus for concern. The progressive increase in concerns and challenges related to antibiotic resistance has been felt globally, with many campaigns developed by several societies and government agencies to promote more prudent prescribing, reduce unnecessary antibiotic use, and increase surveillance and detection of emerging resistance patterns within hospitals and their surrounding communities.[3–5,14–16] In the United States,

major steps were put into motion approximately a decade ago by the CDC with initiatives to decrease antibiotic prescribing (especially for upper respiratory tract infections that are often caused by viruses) and by the Food and Drug Administration with changes in approved product labeling with most antibiotics that attempt to address optimal antibiotic use.[3,4]

Despite all of the publicity in the medical literature and in the lay press (including the Internet) about antibiotic resistance concerns, the true "wake up call" in dermatology came with the emergence of skin infections caused by community-acquired methicillin-resistant *S aureus*. Once community-acquired methicillin-resistant *S aureus* surfaced in the United States, skin infections caused by methicillin-resistant *S aureus* were seen by dermatologists in their offices on a daily basis, or at least several times each week or month. Having these cases in front of them on a regular basis, and seeing first hand cutaneous infections cause by strains of *S aureus* that are resistant to commonly used antibiotics (penicillins, cephalosporins, macrolides, clindamycin) brought greater attention among dermatologists to the clinical relevance of antibiotic resistance beyond just the hospital environment. Nevertheless, many questions remain within the general dermatology community regarding how the use of topical and oral antibiotics by dermatologists contributes to the overall impact of antibiotic resistance and whether the resistance patterns that are created are truly relevant clinically.

The first dedicated group within dermatology in the United States to formally address the subject of antibiotic use and the potential implications of antibiotic resistance in dermatology is the Scientific Panel on Antibiotic Use in Dermatology, formed in 2005.[2–4] Over time, additional initiatives have been brought forward within the United States and globally by dermatology groups (eg, Global Alliance) and by pharmaceutical companies.[5,9,17,18] Much more data are needed in this subject area, because many questions still remain. This article summarizes important principles gleaned from the continued efforts of the Scientific Panel on Antibiotic Use in Dermatology; other groups who are working diligently in this area, such as the CDC and the Canadian Antimicrobial Resistance Alliance; and from the published literature.

MAJOR PREMISE #2: THE IMPORTANCE OF ANTIBIOTIC RESISTANCE IN DERMATOLOGY EXTENDS FAR BEYOND *PROPIONIBACTERIUM ACNES*

Principle #4: Administration of antibiotics systemically or topically causes "ecologic mischief" with collateral damage related to antibiotic resistance that is often underappreciated in the clinical setting. Antibiotic use induces the emergence of less sensitive bacterial strains among exposed commensal and transient flora, including pathogenic bacteria, through antibiotic selection pressure.

Principle #5: Systemically administered antibiotics expose bacteria present on skin and within mucosal tracts leading to the emergence of less sensitive bacterial strains and changes in the microbiome.

Principle #6: Topical antibiotics applied to facial skin induce the emergence of less sensitive bacterial strains present at the site of application, at remote skin sites where the antibiotic has not been applied, and with an increase in nasal staphylococcal carriage.

Principle #7: Resistant strains that emerge subsequent to use of an antibiotic can persist for several weeks to months after discontinuation of therapy.

In dermatology, the progressive increase in antibiotic-resistant *Propionibacterium acnes* has been well established, outwardly discussed for several years, and has been shown to reduce the efficacy of therapy for AV.[3–5,17–27] However, it has been difficult for dermatologists to appreciate the clinical relevance of antibiotic-resistant *P acnes* because the use of combination regimens with other agents (eg, benzoyl peroxide [BP], topical retinoids) for AV results in improvement in most patients. Data showing that concomitant use of BP reduces the quantity and emergence of antibiotic-resistant *P acnes* strains at skin sites where BP is applied (ie, face) has created some comfort level with antibiotic use for AV. However, these data do not address antibiotic exposure at skin sites where BP is not applied, potential resistance patterns among bacteria other than *P acnes*, and resistance patterns within the oropharyngeal (OP), gastrointestinal (GI), and genitourinary/vaginal (GU-V) tracts.[3,5–7,17–27]

Because they do not encounter the clinical sequelae of infections occurring at sites other than skin, many dermatologists have difficulty appreciating the "ecologic mischief" or "collateral damage" that oral and topical antibiotics can create by inducing resistance through antibiotic selection pressure. Selection pressure increases the emergence and quantity of bacteria that are less sensitive to the antibiotic among the normal commensal and transient flora on the skin, and within the bacterial population of the OP, GI, and GU-V tracts that are exposed to systemic (ie, oral) antibiotic therapy.[1–4,6,11,17] Notably, topical antibiotic use on the face can induce antibiotic-

resistant organisms (ie, staphylococci) on remote skin sites (eg, the back) and within the anterior nares.[23,27] It is hard for many individuals to comprehend or accept that the antibiotic-resistant bacteria that develop when antibiotics are used to treat a disorder, such as AV, may be clinically relevant because they can potentially contribute to another type of infection in the individual or in others who the organisms may be spread to at a later time. At minimum, it has been established that use of oral and/or topical antibiotics for treatment of AV significantly increases OP streptococcal colonization and selects for a greater quantity of antibiotic-resistant strains.[17,18,27,28] It has been shown that after discontinuation of an oral antibiotic, resistant strains that emerge can persists for weeks to months.[29,30]

MAJOR PREMISE #3: MEASURES TO REDUCE ANTIBIOTIC EXPOSURE CONTRIBUTE TO REDUCED PREVALENCE OF ANTIBIOTIC-RESISTANT BACTERIA

Principle #8. When treating AV with an oral antibiotic, concomitant topical therapy is indicated. It is strongly recommended that antibiotic monotherapy not be used to treat AV.

Principle #9. When treating AV with an oral antibiotic, it is optimal to combine with a rational topical regimen. It is highly favorable to include BP as a part of the topical regimen to reduce the proliferation and emergence of resistant P acnes *strains.*

Principle #10. When starting an oral antibiotic agent to treat AV, it is important for the clinician to prepare an exit strategy for the discontinuation of antibiotic therapy, using an optimized topical regimen to sustain suppression of acne lesion development. Topical retinoid therapy and also the combination of BP and a topical retinoid have been shown to maintain reasonable remission of acne after discontinuation of oral antibiotic therapy.

Oral and topical antibiotics are to be used for AV as part of a combination therapy approach that includes a topical regimen, preferably inclusive of a BP formulation that has been shown to adequately reduce the magnitude of *P acnes* skin colonization.[3,4,6,7,23,24] However, this does not address prevention of resistance of *P acnes* present at sites where BP is not applied, nor does this address exposure of the microbiome present within the GI, OP, or GU-V tracts to antibiotics that are administered systemically. In addition, whether or not BP reduces the emergence of antibiotic resistance among bacteria other than *P acnes* (eg, staphylococci, streptococci) has not been studied. Therefore, even with best efforts to reduce emergence of antibiotic-resistant bacteria during treatment of AV that includes antibiotic therapy, it is not possible to fully avert the emergence of bacteria that are less sensitive to the administered antibiotic.

When oral antibiotics are administered in combination with a rational topical regimen for AV, how long is the oral antibiotic to be prescribed? Unfortunately, data are relatively limited. Nevertheless, there are studies that address topical maintenance therapy to control AV after discontinuation of oral doxycycline in patients with moderate AV and severe AV that responded favorably to initial combination treatment with a topical regimen and oral doxycycline over the first 3 months.[31–33] These studies evaluated maintenance phases of 3 months with adapalene 0.1% gel once daily, 4 months with tazarotene 0.1% cream once daily, or 6 months with adapalene 0.1%–BP 2.5% gel once daily, with favorable outcomes noted in many subjects. Importantly, an effective and well-tolerated topical retinoid is an important component of maintenance therapy for AV. Nevertheless, topical maintenance therapy is not adequate in all patients, with many requiring reinstitution of oral antibiotic therapy, or use of an alternative therapy, such as oral isotretinoin or a physical modality.[6,7]

Based on the data available with AV, it seems that as a general rule after 3 to 4 months of compliant oral antibiotic use in combination with a topical regimen, the oral antibiotic may be stopped provided that at least a greater than or equal to 50% overall improvement in AV has been observed, especially with inflammatory lesions.[6,31–33] Undoubtedly, some patients may warrant a longer course depending on the severity of AV at baseline and their level of adherence. When the response is not adequate, poor adherence may be a major factor, or the oral antibiotic prescribed may not be effective in that patient, necessitating use of an alternative approach.

Principle #11: Unlike AV, which involves a specific bacterium as a component of the pathophysiology, rosacea has not been shown to be associated with the need to reduce a specific bacterium. Multiple studies have shown that many cases of papulopustular rosacea may be treated effectively with subantimicrobial dosing of doxycycline.

Unlike AV, where reduction in a bacterium (*P acnes*) has been correlated with therapeutic benefit, the pathophysiology of rosacea has not been shown to be associated with a bacterial component that is linked directly with the pathogenesis of rosacea.[34–41] Although not completely understood, the pathophysiology of rosacea seems to involve inflammatory pathways, some of which can be inhibited or down-regulated by tetracycline agents, especially doxycycline and minocycline.[34–40] Based on several studies that have evaluated anti-inflammatory versus antibiotic dose-response and specific formulations, the only tetracycline agent able to achieve anti-inflammatory activity without inducing antibiotic selection pressure is doxycycline. The microbiologic data supporting the lack of emergence of antibiotic resistance associated with subantimicrobial doxycycline evaluated use versus placebo over prolonged durations of 6 to 18 months, and included microbiologic assessments from mouth, skin, GI tract, and vaginal tract.[1,38–45] Subantimicrobial dosing of doxycycline has been well-documented with a specific 40-mg modified-release capsule formulation administered once daily (Doxy-MR 40 mg; Oracea 40-mg capsules, Galderma Laboratories, Fort Worth, TX) and with immediate-release 20-mg tablets administered twice daily. There are several studies and case report series that substantiate the clinical efficacy and safety of subantimicrobial dosing of doxycycline, primarily for treatment of papulopustular rosacea, but also for AV and perioral dermatitis.[42–51]

Principle #12: Recent systemic antibiotic exposure can affect therapeutic outcomes when treating bacterial infections.

Although the emergence of antibiotic resistance is well established after administration of antibiotic therapy, there is little hard evidence demonstrating that use of an oral antibiotic for AV creates antibiotic resistance patterns that are clinically relevant and apparent in "real world" practice.

Although not reported specifically from use of antibiotics in dermatology, it has been shown in a population-based surveillance study (N = 3339) using multivariate analysis that in patients who present with pneumococcal pneumonia, the likelihood of pneumococcal resistance to an antibiotic is markedly increased if the patient had received that antibiotic within the 3 months before presentation.[52] For example, exposure to azithromycin within 3 months before presentation resulted in a 9.93-fold greater risk of infection with macrolide (erythromycin)-resistant *Streptococcus pneumonia* and fluoroquinolone exposure within 3 months before presentation resulted in a 12.1-fold greater risk of infection with levofloxacin-resistant *S pneumonia*.[52] These data provide some evidence that at least recent antibiotic use can influence bacterial resistance patterns that may be clinically relevant with the potential to affect therapeutic outcomes when treating infections.[52]

The reverse perspective is also important to keep in mind because the prevalence of antibiotic resistance can be favorably modified over time by decreasing overall antibiotic exposure within geographic communities.[3,4,11,19,53–55] There is good evidence gleaned from data collected in several countries to support that reduced prescribing of a given antibiotic correlates directly with a decrease in the magnitude of antibiotic resistance in the community.[56–58] One report showed that the prevalence of bacterial resistance to macrolide antibiotics decreased in direct correlation with a reduction in the number of macrolide prescriptions written per capita in the community.[58]

MAJOR PREMISE #4: SOME CLINICAL SITUATIONS WHERE ANTIBIOTICS ARE OFTEN ROUTINELY PRESCRIBED WARRANT RECONSIDERATION BECAUSE ANTIBIOTIC THERAPY IS USUALLY NOT NEEDED

Principle #13: Available data suggest that routine use of antibiotic therapy is not recommended as a treatment of inflamed epidermal cysts, as prophylactic perioperative treatment with office-based dermatologic surgical procedures, and as treatment of chronic leg ulcers.

Inflamed epidermal cysts are commonly encountered in clinical practice. Associated inflammation occurs when subcutaneous rupture of the cyst wall occurs and its spilled contents induce the equivalent of a "foreign body reaction" in the dermis and upper subcutis.[59] When the magnitude of this inflammation is brisk, the affected site becomes visibly inflamed with an expanded area of lesional and perilesional erythema and suffusion that may be warm to touch, is often tender, and is easily misdiagnosed as a bacterial abscess. A study of inflamed epidermal cysts showed an absence of bacterial infection in most cases.[59] Indeed, it may be difficult to distinguish between an inflamed epidermal cyst and an abscess caused by bacterial infection. However, an incision and drainage procedure (I&D) is indicated when a bacterial abscess or inflamed epidermal cyst are suspected clinically. Content expression/removal during I&D usually reveals at least partial fragments of an epidermal cyst if this is the cause. In cases where bacterial infection is suspected clinically, a bacterial culture with sensitivity testing may help direct antibiotic therapy if infection is confirmed and I&D alone is not deemed to be adequate based on clinical evaluation.[60] Overall, oral antibiotic use has been reported to be unnecessary in the absence of documented infection by a bacterial pathogen.[61]

Another scenario where antibiotics are often used routinely despite a lack of evidence supporting their benefit is prophylactic use before and after common office-based dermatologic procedures, especially in patients who are immunocompetent and at very low risk for bacterial infection.[61]

Such procedures include biopsies, shave/saucerization procedures, excisions, and closures. Available data support a very low infection rate with such procedures when performed in an ambulatory setting. Prophylactic antibiotic therapy is only warranted in specific circumstances among high-risk patients or when the surgical procedure extends beyond skin into mucosal regions (ie, mouth, nose). Application of a topical antibiotic to the surgical site as part of postoperative wound care or for treatment of chronic leg ulcers has not been shown to be helpful overall in preventing infection, but can sometimes select for more virulent bacterial pathogens, and may be associated with allergic contact dermatitis (eg, bacitracin, neomycin).[61]

REFERENCES

1. Kim S, Michaels BD, Kim GK, et al. Systemic antimicrobial agents. In: Wolverton SE, editor. Comprehensive dermatologic therapy. 3rd edition. Philadephia (PA): Saunders-Elsevier; 2013. p. 61–97.
2. Sanchez G, Del Rosso JQ, Leyden JJ, et al. Scientific panel on antibiotic therapy update. J Clin Aesthet Dermatol, in press.
3. Del Rosso JQ, Leyden JJ, Thiboutot D, et al. Antibiotic use in acne vulgaris and rosacea: clinical considerations and resistance issues of significance to dermatologists. Cutis 2008;82(2 Suppl 2):5–12.
4. Leyden JJ, Del Rosso JQ, Webster GF. Clinical considerations in the treatment of acne vulgaris and other inflammatory skin disorders: focus on antibiotic resistance. Cutis 2007;79(Suppl 6):9–25.
5. Dreno B, Thiboutot D, Gollnick H, et al. Antibiotic stewardship in dermatology: limiting antibiotic use in acne. Eur J Dermatol 2014;24(3):330–4.
6. Del Rosso JQ, Kim G. Optimizing use of oral antibiotics in acne vulgaris. Dermatol Clin 2009;27(1): 33–42.
7. Gollnick H, Cunliffe W, Berson D, et al. Management of acne: report from a global alliance to improve outcomes in acne. J Am Acad Dermatol 2003; 49(1):S1–37.
8. Strauss JS, Krowchuk DP, Leyden JJ, et al. Guidelines of care for acne management. J Am Acad Dermatol 2007;56(4):651–63.
9. Thiboutout D, Dreno B, Gollnick H, et al. A call to limit antibiotic use in acne. J Drugs Dermatol 2013; 12(12):1331–2.

10. Del Rosso JQ, Baldwin H, Webster G, et al. American Acne and Rosacea Society rosacea medical management guidelines. J Drugs Dermatol 2008; 7(6):531–3.

11. Del Rosso JQ, Leyden JJ. Status report on antibiotic resistance: implications for the dermatologist. Dermatol Clin 2007;25(2):127–32.

12. Rosen T. Antibiotic resistance: an editorial review with recommendations. J Drugs Dermatol 2011; 10(7):724–33.

13. Bradley JS, Guidos R, Baragona S, et al. Anti-infective research and development: problems, challenges, and solutions. Lancet Infect Dis 2007;7(1): 68–78.

14. Sabtu N, Enoch DA, Brown NM. Antibiotic resistance: what, why, where, when, and how? Br Med Bull 2015;116(1):105–13.

15. Klepser ME, Adams AJ, Klepser DG, et al. Antimicrobial stewardship in outpatient settings: leveraging innovative physician-pharmacist collaborations to reduce antibiotic resistance. Health Secur 2015;13(3):166–73.

16. Loo LW, Liew YX, Lee W, et al. Impact of antimicrobial stewardship program (ASP) on outcomes in patients with acute bacterial skin and skin structure infections (ABSSSIs) in an acute-tertiary care hospital. Infect Dis Ther 2015;4(Suppl 1):15–25.

17. Levy RM, Huang EY, Rolling D, et al. Effect of antibiotics on the oropharyngeal flora in patients with acne. Arch Dermatol 2003;139:467–71.

18. Harkaway KS, McGinley KJ, Foglia AN, et al. Antibiotic resistance patterns in coagulase-negative staphylococci after treatment with topical erythromycin, benzoyl peroxide, and combination therapy. Br J Dermatol 1992;126:585–90.

19. Eady AH, Cove JH, Layton AM. Is antibiotic resistance in cutaneous propionibacteria clinically relevant? Implications of resistance for acne patients and prescribers. Am J Clin Dermatol 2003;12:813–31.

20. Cooper AJ. Systemic review of Propionibacterium acnes resistance to systemic antibiotics. Med J Aust 1998;169:259–61.

21. Mills O, Thornsberry C, Cardin CW, et al. Bacterial resistance and therapeutic outcome following three months of topical acne therapy with 2% erythromycin gel versus its vehicle. Acta Derm Venereol 2002;82:260–5.

22. Eady EA, Cove JH, Holland KT, et al. Erythromycin resistant propionibacteria in antibiotic treated acne patients: association with therapeutic failure. Br J Dermatol 1989;121:51–7.

23. Tanghettti E, Popp KF. A current review of topical benzoyl peroxide: new perspectives on formulation and utilization. Dermatol Clin 2009;27:17–24.

24. Cunliffe WJ, Holland KT, Bojar R, et al. A randomized, double-blind comparison of a clindamycin phosphate/benzoyl peroxide gel formulation and a matching clindamycin gel with respect to microbiologic activity and clinical efficacyin the topical treatment of acne vulgaris. Clin Ther 2002; 24:1117–33.

25. Leyden JJ, Del Rosso JQ. The effect of benzoyl peroxide 9.8% emollient foam on reduction of Propionibacterium acnes on the back using a short contact therapy approach. J Drugs Dermatol 2012; 11(7):830–3.

26. Leyden JJ, Preston N, Osborn C, et al. In-vivo effectiveness of adapalene 0.1%/benzoyl peroxide 2.5% gel on antibiotic-sensitive and resistant Propionibacterium acnes. J Clin Aesthet Dermatol 2011;4(5):22–6.

27. Bowe W, Leyden JJ. Clinical implications of antibiotic resistance risk: risk of systemic infection from Staphylococcus and Streptococcus. In: Shalita AR, Del Rosso JQ, Webster GF, editors. Acne vulgaris. New York: Informa Healthcare; 2011. p. 125–33.

28. Margolis DJ, Bowe WP, Hoffstad O, et al. Antibiotic treatment of acne may be associated with upper respiratory tract infections. Arch Dermatol 2005; 141:1132–6.

29. Malhotra-Kumar S, Lammens C, Coenen S, et al. The effect of azithromycin and clarithromycin therapy on pharyngeal carriage of macrolide-resistant streptococci in healthy volunteers: a ramdomized, double blind, placebo-controlled study. Lancet 2007;369(9560):482–90.

30. Berg HF, Tjhie JHT, Scheffer GJ, et al. Emergence and persistence of macrolide resistance in oropharyngeal flora and elimination of nasal carriage of Staphylococcus aureus after therapy with slow-release clarithromycin: a randomized, double-blind, placebo-controlled study. Antimicrob Ag Chemother 2004;48(11):4183–8.

31. Thiboutot DM, Shalita AR, Yamauchi PS, et al. Adapalene gel 0.1% as maintenance therapy for acne vulgaris: a randomized, controlled, investigator-blinded, follow-up of a recent combination study. Arch Dermatol 2006;142(5):597–602.

32. Leyden JJ, Thiboutot DM, Shalita AR, et al. Comparison of tazarotene and minocycline maintenance therapies in acne vulgaris: a multicenter, double-blind, randomized, parallel-group study. Arch Dermatol 2006;142(5):605–12.

33. Poulin Y, Sanchez NP, Bucko A, et al. A 6-month maintenance therapy with adapalene-benzoyl peroxide gel prevents and continuously improves efficacy among patients with severe acne vulgaris: results of a randomized controlled trial. Br J Dermatol 2011;164(6):1376–82.

34. Crawford GH, Pelle MT, James WD. Rosacea: I. Etiology, pathogenesis, and subtype classification. J Am Acad Dermatol 2004;51:327–41.

35. Yamasaki K, Gallo RL. The molecular pathology of rosacea. J Dermatol Sci 2009;55:77–81.

36. Steinhoff M, Buddenkotte J, Aubert J, et al. Clinical, cellular, and molecular aspects in the pathophysiology of rosacea. J Investig Dermatol Symp Proc 2011;15:2–11.

37. Del Rosso JQ. Advances in understanding and managing rosacea, part 1: connecting the dots between pathophysiological mechanisms and common clinical features of rosacea with emphasis on vascular changes and facial erythema. J Clin Aesthet Dermatol 2012;5(3):16–25.

38. Korting HC, Schöllmann C. Tetracycline actions relevant to rosacea treatment. Skin Pharmacol Physiol 2009;22:287–94.

39. Del Rosso JQ. Update on rosacea pathogenesis and correlation with medical therapeutic agents. Cutis 2006;78:97–100.

40. Kennedy Carney C, Cantrell W, Elewski BE. Rosacea: a review of current topical, systemic and light based therapies. G Ital Dermatol Venereol 2009; 144:673–88.

41. Lazaridou E, Giannopoulou C, Fotiadou C, et al. The potential role of microorganisms in the development of rosacea. J Dtsch Dermatol Ges 2011;9:21–5.

42. Skidmore R, Kovach R, Walker C, et al. Effects of subantimicrobial-dose doxycycline in the treatment of moderate acne. Arch Dermatol 2003;139(4):459–64.

43. Del Rosso JQ, Webster GW, Jackson M, et al. Two randomized phase II clinical trials evaluating anti-inflammatory dose doxycycline (40-mg doxycycline, USP capsules) administered once daily for treatment of rosacea. J Am Acad Dermatol 2007;56: 791–801.

44. Preshaw PM, Novak MJ, Mellonig J, et al. Modified-release subantimicrobial dose doxycycline enhances scaling and root planing in subjects with periodontal disease. J Periodontol 2008;79(3):440–52.

45. Del Rosso JQ. Anti-inflammatory dose doxycycline in the treatment of rosacea. J Drugs Dermatol 2009;8:664–8.

46. Webster GF. An open-label, community-based, 12-week assessment of the effectiveness and safety of monotherapy with doxycycline 40 mg (30-mg immediate-release and 10-mg delayed-release beads). Cutis 2010;86(5 Suppl):7–15.

47. Baldwin H. A community-based study of the effectiveness of doxycycline 40 mg (30-mg immediate-release and 10-mg delayed-release beads) on quality of life and satisfaction with treatment in participants with rosacea. Cutis 2010;86(5 Suppl):26–36.

48. Del Rosso JQ. Effectiveness and safety of doxycycline 40 mg (30-mg immediate-release and 10-mg delayed-release beads) once daily as add-on therapy to existing topical regimens for the treatment of papulopustular rosacea: results from a community-based trial. Cutis 2010;86(5 Suppl):16–25.

49. Fowler JF Jr. Combined effect of anti-inflammatory dose doxycycline (40-mg doxycycline, USP monohydrate controlled-release capsules) and metronidazole topical gel 1% in the treatment of rosacea. J Drugs Dermatol 2007;6:641–5.

50. Moore A, Ling M, Bucko A, et al. Efficacy and safety of subantimicrobial dose, modified-release doxycycline 40 mg versus doxycycline 100 mg versus placebo for the treatment of inflammatory lesions in moderate and severe acne: a randomized, double-blinded, controlled study. J Drugs Dermatol 2015; 14(6):581–6.

51. Del Rosso JQ. Management of papulopustular rosacea and perioral dermatitis with emphasis on iatrogenic causation or exacerbation of inflammatory facial dermatoses: use of doxycycline-modified release 40 mg capsule once daily in combination with properly selected skin care as an effective therapeutic approach. J Clin Aesthet Dermatol 2011;4(8):20–30.

52. Vanderkooi OG, Low DE, Green K, et al. Predicting antimicrobial resistance in invasive pneumococcal infections. Clin Infect Dis 2005;40(9):1288–97.

53. Del Rosso JQ. Update from the scientific panel on antibiotic use in dermatology: clinical considerations for the dermatologist. Cutis 2008;82(2 Suppl 2):3–4.

54. Ross JI, Snelling AM, Eady EA, et al. Phenotypic and genotypic characterization of antibiotic-resistant Propionibacterium acnes isolated from acne patients attending dermatology clinics in Europe, the U.S.A., Japan, and Australia. Br J Dermatol 2001; 144(2):339–46.

55. Ross JI, Snelling AM, Carnegie E, et al. Antibiotic-resistant acne: lessons from Europe. Br J Dermatol 2003;148(3):467–78.

56. Seppala H, Klaukka T, Vuopio-Varkila J, et al. The effect of changes in the consumption of macrolide antibiotics on erythromycin resistance in group A streptococci in Finland. Finish Study Group for Antimicrobial Resistance. N Engl J Med 1997;337(7):441–6.

57. Sakata H. The change of macrolide resistance rates in group A Streptococcus isolates from children between 2002 and 2013 in Asahikawa city. J Infect Chemother 2015;21(5):398–401.

58. Bergman M, Huikko S, Pihlajamaki M, et al. Effect of macrolide consumption on erythromycin resistance in Streptococcus pyogenes in Finland in 1997-2001. Clin Infect Dis 2004;38(9):1251–6.

59. Diven DG, Dozier SE, Meyer DJ, et al. Bacteriology of inflamed and uninflamed epidermal inclusion cysts. Arch Dermatol 1998;134(1):49–51.

60. Fahimi J, Singh A, Frazee BW. The role of adjunctive antibiotics in the treatment of skin and soft tissue abscesses: a systematic review and meta-analysis. CJEM 2015;17(4):420–32.

61. Hirschmann JV. When antibiotics are unnecessary. Dermatol Clin 2009;27(1):75–83.

Oral Isotretinoin
New Developments Relevant to Clinical Practice

 CrossMark

Jerry Tan, MD, FRCPC[a,b,]*, Sanwarjit Boyal, BMSc[c],
Karishma Desai, BMSc[d], Sanja Knezevic, BSc[d]

KEYWORDS

- Isotretinoin • Acne • Dosing • Relapse • Adverse events • Mechanism

KEY POINTS

- Isotretinoin has multiple mechanisms of action in acne, including sebocyte apoptosis, inhibition of toll-like receptor 2, and suppression of certain hormones implicated in pathogenesis.
- With increasing acne severity, higher cumulative doses of isotretinoin are required to achieve clearance.
- There is no moderate-grade or high-grade evidence supporting the cumulative isotretinoin dose range of 120 to 150 mg/kg.
- Depression and suicidal risk are associated with acne; isotretinoin may confer a slight increase in depression risk.
- Recommendations to avoid acne scar repair procedures within 6 months after isotretinoin should be reconsidered.

INTRODUCTION

Since its introduction 3.5 decades ago, oral isotretinoin has been the single most effective treatment of acne.[1] Although its potential for side effects and monitoring requirements restrict its use, it has resulted in profound improvement in the lives of the patients treated. Nevertheless, this medication continues to be controversial regarding the potential for an array of adverse effects and the risk of birth defects. Although there are multiple recent reviews on oral isotretinoin in the literature, most focus on the pregnancy risk and pregnancy prevention programs; mental health disorders, including depression and suicidal risk; and bowel disease.[2–6] Aside from considerations of risk, there have also been advances in the use of this medication to enhance tolerability while maintaining effectiveness, measures to enhance bioavailability, clarification of the outcomes of different dosing routines and cumulative threshold dosing, and other evidence-based applications for the use of this medication. This article focuses on these advances to provide a perspective on dosing considerations relevant to maximize improvement while minimizing the potential for harms. Specifically, the objective is to provide a practical update relevant to clinical

Funding: None.
Conflicts of Interest: J. Tan has been an advisor and/or speaker and has received grants and/or honoraria from Roche and Cipher Pharmaceuticals. The other authors have no conflicts to declare.
[a] Schulich School of Medicine and Dentistry, Western University, Windsor Campus, Medical Education Building, 401 Sunset Ave, Windsor, Ontario N9B3P4, Canada; [b] Windsor Clinical Research Inc., 2224 Walker Road, Suite 300B, Windsor, Ontario N8W5L7, Canada; [c] Windsor Clinical Research Inc., 2224 Walker Road, Suite 300B, Windsor, Ontario N8W5L7, Canada; [d] Department of Medicine, Schulich School of Medicine and Dentistry, Western University, Windsor Campus, Medical Education Building, 401 Sunset Ave, Windsor, Ontario N9B3P4, Canada
* Corresponding author. 2224 Walker Road, Suite 300, Windsor, Ontario N8W5L7, Canada.
E-mail addresses: jerrytan@wcri.ca; jerrytan@bellnet.ca

Dermatol Clin 34 (2016) 175–184
http://dx.doi.org/10.1016/j.det.2015.11.002
0733-8635/16/$ – see front matter © 2016 Elsevier Inc. All rights reserved.

derm.theclinics.com

practice in the use of oral isotretinoin, including new findings regarding mechanism of action; means to enhance bioavailability, including a new formulation of oral isotretinoin; dosimetry to optimize acne clearance while minimizing the risk of avoidable adverse events; evidence regarding cumulative threshold dosing of oral isotretinoin 120 to 150 mg/kg; and current information on the timing of scar correction procedures after isotretinoin treatment.

Mechanism of Action

Isotretinoin, the cis-isomer of transretinoic acid, is converted in vivo to all-trans retinoic acid. The latter is the active effector molecule inducing cellular effects via binding to nuclear retinoic acid receptors, retinoid X receptors (RXRs), and retinoid acid receptors (RARs).[7] The pathogenic mechanisms of acne involve sebum hypersecretion, intraductal epithelial hyperkeratinization, Propionibacterium acnes proliferation, and inflammation. Although isotretinoin has been shown to affect these pathogenic factors, only recently have the mechanisms been understood.

Isotretinoin has been shown to have direct effects on sebocytes, leading to sebum suppression, and on inflammation by inhibiting innate immune system activation. In sebocytes, isotretinoin induces cell cycle arrest and apoptosis by a mechanism independent of RAR binding. This effect likely contributes to its sebosuppressive activity and ameliorative effect on acne.[8] Sebocyte apoptosis was shown to be mediated by tumor necrosis factor–related apoptosis-inducing ligand[9] and neutrophil gelatinase-associated lipocalin (NGAL).[10] The latter functions in innate immune defense against gram-negative bacteria. In patients with acne treated with isotretinoin, increased skin surface NGAL levels have been observed; an effect that precedes sebum suppression and reduction in P acnes.[11] It is speculated that reduction in the level of P acnes may be caused by the combined effect of these outcomes.

Peripheral blood monocytes from patients with acne have been shown to express higher levels of toll-like receptor 2 (TLR-2) and show greater expression of TLR-2 following exposure to P acnes. Isotretinoin at 1 week reduced monocyte TLR-2 expression and inflammatory cytokine release induced by P acnes. Note that this effect persisted to 6 months posttreatment, implying that TLR-2 modulation may be involved in the long-term therapeutic response to isotretinoin.[12]

Recently, oral isotretinoin was found to result in significant changes in various hormones, including some implicated in acne pathogenesis, such as insulin-like growth factor 1 and growth hormone, in a dose-dependent manner. In 105 patients with acne divided into 3 isotretinoin dosing groups (0.5–1 mg/kg/d, 0.2–0.5 mg/kg/d, and intermittent 0.5–1 mg/kg/d for 1 week per month) hormone levels were measured at 3 months. Levels of luteinizing hormone, prolactin, total testosterone, adrenocorticotropic hormone, cortisol, insulin-like growth factor 1, growth hormone, and free T3 and T4 were reduced, whereas levels of dehydroepiandrosterone sulfate increased. The greatest effects were seen with the highest of the 3 dose regimens (0.5–1 mg/kg/d). The smallest effect was observed for the intermittent dosing of 0.5 to 1 mg/kg/d for 1 week per month. Although the investigators suggested that changes in some of these hormone levels may be one of the mechanisms of action of isotretinoin in acne, some of these effects may also contribute to potential adverse effects, particularly because most treatment courses extend beyond 3 months.[13] Further study of these hormonal changes is a priority.

Enhancing Bioavailability

Isotretinoin, a derivative of vitamin A, is highly lipophilic and bioavailability is enhanced with fat coingestion. Hence the standard practice recommendation of ingestion with food, particularly a high-fat meal, to enhance absorption. Initial pharmacokinetic studies of oral isotretinoin involved ingestion of a standardized high-fat meal comprising 1000 calories with 50% from fat.[14] The bioavailability of standard oral isotretinoin formulations is approximately 60% lower in fasted conditions than after fatty meals, as described earlier.[15]

It is inconceivable that such a meal will be taken on a daily basis by patients on oral isotretinoin in usual practice. Thus, recommendations in standard practice for coingestion of oral isotretinoin include foods with high fat content (Table 1). Almost 1 in 3 adolescents do not have breakfast.[16] Thus, inconsistent eating habits and inadequate fat content of coingestants may result in suboptimal and varying bioavailability.

A related issue is that the standard for bioequivalence of generic formulations is 80% to 125% of the innovator product Accutane (Roche Laboratories). Immediately before and for 2 decades after its approval for use in the United States in 1982, studies on dosing in acne clearance and potential for remission were done with the innovator, generic formulations being available in the United States only since 2002.[17] If a cumulative threshold dose, as recommended by other investigators, is used as a therapeutic end point, there is a potential for underdosing while using generics.[18]

Table 1
Foods to consider for coingestion with oral isotretinoin

Food/Beverage	Calories (kcal)	Fat (g)	Fat Content by Calories (%)
Standardized high-fat meal[14]: 2 eggs, fried in butter, 2 strips of bacon, 2 slices of toast with butter, hash browns (220 g) and milk (240 mL)	1000	56	50
Cup of whole milk	149	8	48
Tablespoon of peanut butter	94 (31/teaspoon)	8	76
Tablespoon of olive oil	119 (40/teaspoon)	14	100
Pork chop	265	15	50
Pizza slice	280	13	40
Steak (85 g)	190	8	36
Fried chicken drumstick	193	16	53
California avocado (1 fruit)	227	29	83
Whole egg (1, large)	72	5	60
Dark chocolate (1 bar)	604	43	64

Data from US Department of Agriculture (USDA): Agricultural Research Service. National nutrient database for standard reference release 27. Available at: http://ndb.nal.usda.gov/. Accessed March 07, 2015.

Efficacy

The most rigorous studies regarding isotretinoin efficacy and adverse events in acne are from large randomized trials designed to minimize risk of bias. Within the constraints of that framework, only 2 studies over the past decade provide evidence on the potential of oral isotretinoin in achieving global success in acne.

In a noninferiority study of conventional oral isotretinoin versus oral isotretinoin-Lidose, the total cumulative dose attained was 126 mg/kg. Although the primary outcome was reduction in nodule counts on the face and trunk, information on rates of complete/almost complete clearance was also available. The proportions of subjects achieving complete/almost complete clearance with conventional oral isotretinoin and with isotretinoin-Lidose were 89% and 84%, respectively.[19] A more recent study in severe nodular acne compared the relative efficacy and tolerability of oral doxycycline 200 mg daily plus fixed-dose adapalene 0.1%/benzoyl peroxide 2.5% gel with conventional oral isotretinoin.[20] The resultant cumulative dose was also 126 mg/kg and the proportion of subjects attaining clear/almost clear facial acne in the oral isotretinoin arm was 77% (data on file, Galderma). For both studies, facial acne was not clear/almost clear in approximately 10% to 20% at end of treatment in the studies discussed earlier. It can be inferred that more prolonged treatment and correspondingly higher cumulative doses would be required to achieve complete clearance in all patients. Furthermore, these findings applied only to facial

acne. Because truncal acne is known to lag in response to treatment compared to facial acne, it is anticipated that longer treatment durations, and therefore greater cumulative doses, are required for those with truncal involvement. Additional support that higher doses are likely required includes 2 studies in severe acne (**Table 2**): 1 retrospective and another prospective in which the mean cumulative doses required were 290 mg/kg[21] and 264 mg/kg,[22] respectively.

Low and Alternative Dosing Regimens

The past decade has witnessed an increasing number of reports on oral isotretinoin in mild and moderate acne along with alternative dosing.[23–25] Specifically these regimens have been characterized as minidose, comprising 20 mg up to 2 days per week; low dose, with daily dosing of 0.25 to 0.5 mg/kg/d; alternate day; or intermittent dosing, such as 7 or 10 days per month.[25] The potential advantage of these regimens is maintenance of efficacy while reducing adverse events (**Table 3**).[24,26,27]

A recent study showed that improvement was similar for those receiving 0.5 to 0.7 mg/kg/d compared with 0.25 to 0.4 mg/kg/d and both were superior to 0.5 to 0.7 mg/kg/d once daily for 1 of every 4 weeks. Furthermore, relapses (defined as moderate or higher grade of acne) for the daily dosing groups were also similar and statistically superior to the intermittent dosing group. Adverse events were most frequently reported in the higher daily dose group, with cheilitis

Table 2
Recent studies reporting isotretinoin efficacy

Study	N	Trial Design	Severity	Daily Dosing (mg/kg/d)	Treatment Duration	Cumulative Dosing (mg/kg)
Webster et al,[19] 2014	925	Noninferiority, randomized, evaluator blinded	Severe recalcitrant nodular acne	0.5 1	Initial 4 wk Final 16 wk	126
Tan et al,[20] 2014	266	Noninferiority, randomized, evaluator blinded	Severe facial acne	0.5 1	Initial 4 wk Final 16 wk	126
Cyrulnik et al,[21] 2012	80	Retrospective review	Cystic (91.2%) Severe Cystic (8.8%)	Mean = 1.6	178 d	290.1
Blasiak et al,[22] 2013	116	Prospective, observational	Severe nodulocystic acne	Not stated	Mean = 6.3 mo	264

in 94% and xerosis in 31%, compared with the lower daily dose group, with rates of 65% and 6%, respectively.[23] A shortcoming of that study is that an even higher, more conventional 0.7 to 1.0 mg/kg/d dose was not included.

Other studies have shown that lower doses in mild to moderate acne achieve excellent clearance of acne with high rates of remission despite attainment of cumulative doses less than 120 mg/kg. In an open-label prospective study to determine the efficacy of low-dose isotretinoin in inducing clearance and inducing remission of mild and moderate acne, dosing was initiated with 0.2 mg/kg/d and increased by 5 mg every 2 weeks to intolerance; intolerance was not further defined. Patients were treated for an additional month beyond complete acne clearance (mean cumulative dose of isotretinoin, 81 mg/kg) and maintained for 1 year on nightly adapalene 0.1% cream. At 2 years, relapse, defined as severity greater than mild, was observed in 13 of 139 patients (9%).[28]

A recent study on low-grade adult acne showed the efficacy of isotretinoin 5 mg/d in reducing acne lesions and improving quality of life. Improvements in lesion counts were observed by 4 weeks and continued through the 32 weeks of treatment. At that juncture, 62.5% of subjects were completely clear of acne, defined as no acne lesions. Adverse events were primarily mild dryness of the skin and/or mucous membranes (62%) managed with topical moisturizers and lip balm.[29]

Relapse

The initial recommendation of a minimum cumulative dose of 120 mg/kg for oral isotretinoin was

Table 3
Recent studies using low and alternative dosing regimens

Study	N	Trial Design	Severity	Daily Dosing (mg/kg/d)	Treatment Duration (wk)	Cumulative Dosing (mg/kg)
Lee et al,[23] 2011	49	Prospective, randomized controlled trial	Moderate acne	0.5–0.7 0.25–0.4 0.5–0.7 for 1 wk every 4 wk	24	Not stated
Borghi et al,[28] 2011	139	Prospective, noncomparative study	Mild acne (17.27%) Moderate acne (83.73%)	0.2; increased by 5 mg every 2 wk until intolerable	Not stated	80.92
Rademaker et al,[29] 2014	58	Randomized, placebo controlled	Low-grade acne	5 mg/d	32	Not stated

based on observations of a reduced rate of relapse.[30] The upper range of 150 mg/kg was established by a guidelines document indicating no further therapeutic gain with oral isotretinoin beyond that threshold.[31] Subsequently, attainment of a cumulative dose of 120 to 150 mg/kg has been widely recommended as an end point for isotretinoin treatment with the goal of increasing the potential for remission. This axiom is present in the most contemporary of acne guidelines, oral isotretinoin review articles, and even in clinical research studies on new formulations of oral isotretinoin.[7,32–35] Notably, it is absent in the most rigorously developed of current acne practice guidelines.[36]

In a large database study linking medical service and pharmacy from the province of Quebec, Canada, predictors of acne relapse (defined as prescription of an acne medication) after oral isotretinoin were evaluated. The cohort comprised 17,351 first-time isotretinoin users with controls matched to each case.[37] A total of 7100 (41%) subjects experienced an acne relapse (40.9%; 95% confidence interval [CI], 40.4–41.4), with half of this group receiving an acne medication within 59 months after completion of isotretinoin treatment. Of these, 26% required a second course of oral isotretinoin treatment. Male gender, age less than 16 years, urban domicile, isotretinoin cumulative doses less than 2450 mg (for a 70-kg patient, equivalent to 35 mg/kg), and treatment with isotretinoin less than 121 days were significantly associated with acne relapse. A progressive reduction in relapse rates with increasing cumulative doses of isotretinoin was noted such that the adjusted rate ratio of the highest dose range of greater than or equal to 7584 mg (for a 70-kg patient, equivalent to 108 mg/kg) was 0.63 (0.57–0.70) relative to those receiving less than 2450 mg. The follow-up duration of up to 20 years was longer than any prior study and likely reflects the true relapse rate. Although this study provided evidence of greater potential for remission with higher cumulative doses, information on baseline acne severity, daily dosimetry, and specific details on absolute relapse were unavailable. Furthermore, relapse, defined as prescription of acne medication, likely underestimates true acne relapse because some subjects may seek over-the-counter or alternative therapy, not present to their physicians for more treatment, or not fill their prescriptions for acne medication. Thus, an alternative perspective is that the 41% relapse rate may underestimate the true rate because there was inadequate information on acne severity, inadequate cumulative dosing to the recommendation of 120 to 150 mg/kg, and some may have

had refractory acne wherein low-dose intermittent isotretinoin may have been prescribed.

In the observational study of 116 patients with severe nodulocystic acne, relapse rates at 1 year were lower in those receiving 220 mg/kg or more compared with those receiving lower doses (<220 mg/kg), with rates of 47.4% and 26.9%, respectively. Although a relapse rate of 33% was reported at 12-month follow-up, the article indicated that 65% of patients reported having had acne in the prior month. This discrepancy suggests that half the subjects with recurrent acne were not being treated with acne medications. Nonetheless, because physical examination was not performed on follow-up, the 65% recurrence rate reported by patients may be an underestimate. Thus, rate of recurrent acne in this study is likely within the range of 33% (use of prescription medication for acne) and 65% (patient self-report of acne).[22]

A systematic review of the literature from 1980 to 2013 found a lack of high-quality studies supporting the cumulative dose of 120 to 150 mg/kg.[38] On a 4-category scale of evidence quality from very low to high, the highest rated studies were 4 that were rated as moderate quality. Of these, none explicitly evaluated the cumulative dose of 120 to 150 mg/kg in acne relapse. Factors likely contributing to lack of high-quality evidence are inconsistencies in definition of key concepts, including acne clearance; treatment end point and relapse; as well as observational and retrospective study design. Nevertheless, when comparing multiple doses within the same study under controlled conditions, higher cumulative doses have consistently resulted in lesser relapse rates compared with lower doses.

Pregnancy Prevention

Recent investigations in women exposed to oral isotretinoin during pregnancy have provided new information on overall rates of exposure and risk for spontaneous abortions and malformations. In a study of 79 pregnant women referred for teratogen-risk counseling because of a history of isotretinoin exposure, 56 continued pregnancies to term. Of these, there were 11 spontaneous abortions, 44 healthy full-term babies, and 1 with multiple congenital abnormalities treated by therapeutic abortion.[39] In the Netherlands, an exposure rate of 2.5 per 10,000 pregnancies was obtained from a cohort study of approximately 200,000 pregnancies over an 8-year period. In total there were 51 pregnancies exposed to isotretinoin: 45 during pregnancy and 6 within 30 days of discontinuing isotretinoin. An adverse outcome was observed in 5: 3 intrauterine deaths and 2 with major congenital anomalies.[40]

The iPledge program is a computerized risk management system established in the United States in 2008 and requires 2 negative pregnancy tests before starting therapy and the use of 2 forms of contraception 30 days both before initiation of oral isotretinoin and on its cessation.[41] Despite the iPledge program, between 2008 and 2011 there were still 150 women annually who became pregnant while on oral isotretinoin in the United States. A recent retrospective study found suboptimal concomitant rates of isotretinoin and contraceptive use before (29%) and after (32%) iPledge initiation.[41] Adherence to contraception use continues to be an issue. An anonymous survey of 75 women of child-bearing potential who agreed to contraceptive methods or abstinence in iPledge found that of the 39 women who were sexually active, condom use had a noncompliance rate of 29%, whereas there was failure to use 2 forms of contraception in 44%.[42] Of the 21 who chose abstinence, 7 had previously been sexually active, of whom 4 continued to be sexually active during treatment. Thus, even within a highly regulated pregnancy registry, there is evidence of ongoing risk behavior for pregnancy.

Recent studies have also examined contraceptive counseling methods by dermatologists. Interviews with 15 women participating in iPledge found that patients comprehended the adverse effect of isotretinoin on pregnancies and understood the risk of birth defects. Nevertheless, they received less information about effective means of contraception and none were fully informed about the advantages and disadvantages of all contraceptive options. Furthermore, many had misconceptions about highly effective reversible contraceptives such as intrauterine devices and subdermal implants.[43] These methods of long-acting reversible contraception can lead to the same typical-use and perfect-use failure rates and are approved for up to 5 years of use.[43,44]

Mental Health Disorders

The association of oral isotretinoin with depression and suicidal ideation has been addressed in multiple recent reviews.[3,4,45–49] Based on the same body of research evidence, some investigators consider the potential for causality with oral isotretinoin in depression to be controversial,[47,49] unsettled,[48] potentially unresolvable,[44] or strongly supportive.[46,50] Comprehensive reviews of this issue in the literature focus on evidence from multiple perspectives, including temporality, outcomes of dechallenge-rechallenge, class effect

of retinoids, dose responsivity, and biological plausibility. The evidence for biological plausibility comes from brain imaging studies and neurochemical pathways.[46,48,50]

The literature on this association largely comprises case reports and retrospective studies, with few prospective trials. However, assessment of quality in these reviews is exclusively qualitative, none using quasiquantitative literature appraisal methodology.[46,48,50] Of the prospective cohort studies, the 2 largest comprised 600[51] and 700[52] subjects with acne treated with oral isotretinoin. Both showed an identical depression rate of 1%. Of the retrospective studies, the largest was a case-control analysis involving 30,496 subjects. This study was the first to show a significant association between isotretinoin and depression, with a relative risk of 2.68 (CI, 1.10–6.48). Limitations of this study were absence of psychiatric confirmation of depression and inadequate determination of preexisting depression, particularly within the context of those with severe acne.[53]

A subsequent review[45] reported the incidence of major depression in adolescents as 3% to 11%[54] and also highlights that acne is associated with depression or suicide. In the study of 3775 adolescents aged 18 to 19 years, 14% reported substantial acne ("a lot" or "very much" on a 4-category scale). Compared with subjects with no/little acne, suicidal ideation was 2-fold and 3-fold higher in girls and boys, respectively. Mental health problems, including depression, were also associated with substantial acne. Potential confounding with oral isotretinoin was mitigated by the low rate of prescribing in this cohort. The investigators concluded that acne, frequently found in late adolescence, is associated with social and psychological problems. Furthermore, suicidal ideation and depression, associated with acne therapy such as oral isotretinoin, may reflect the burden of substantial acne rather than an effect of medication.[55]

The effect of severe acne as distinct from that of oral isotretinoin was also addressed by a study of 5756 patients with severe acne. Time frames were divided into junctures before, during, and after treatment with isotretinoin. The risk of suicide attempts was found to progressively escalate from 3 years before isotretinoin treatment and remained increased until 6 months posttreatment.[56] Thus severe acne, independent of oral isotretinoin, contributes to an increased risk of depression and suicide.

All patients should be informed about uncommon risk for mood and behavioral changes associated with acne and possibly with oral isotretinoin. A brief practical and validated screening instrument with high sensitivity and specificity for major depressive disorders can be of value in practice, such as the 2-item Patient Health Questionnaire (PHQ-2; Copyright Pfizer Inc).[57,58] In patients with positive screen findings, further evaluation with more specific instruments, such as the 9-item PHQ-9 (Copyright Pfizer Inc)[59] or Hamilton Depression Rating Scale[60] can confirm the diagnosis and provide determination of severity.[61] Further management with the family physician and/or a mental health professional is recommended to develop a strategy for ongoing monitoring and mitigation of mental health risk if oral isotretinoin is prescribed. For these patients, consider initiation with a low starting dose of oral isotretinoin and slow escalation.

Inflammatory Bowel Disease

Before 2013, there were 4 epidemiologic studies and 2 abstracts evaluating the association between oral isotretinoin and inflammatory bowel disease (IBD). Two that were initially performed to address case reports of association provided divergent results: one showing no association,[62] the other showing strong association with ulcerative colitis (UC) but not Crohn disease (CD).[63] However, findings from the latter could not be replicated by a subsequent study controlling for prior oral antibiotic use and acne severity while reducing confounding by oral contraceptive use.[64] Another large epidemiologic study from British Columbia, Canada, found no association between oral isotretinoin and IBD.[65] However, a weak association was detected for both topical acne medications and oral isotretinoin with IBD in young subjects (aged 12–19 years), suggesting that the association may be with acne itself rather than its treatment.

Three recent studies also do not show an association of IBD with oral isotretinoin exposure. In a study evaluating risk of IBD in women of reproductive age with use of isotretinoin using a health claims database, the adjusted relative risk for UC was 1.10 (95% CI, 0.44–2.70) and for CD was 0.91 (95% CI, 0.37–2.25).[64] A French National Health Insurance case-control study involving 7593 cases of IBD found no association between oral isotretinoin and UC. Odds ratio (OR) for UC was 1.36 (95% CI, 0.76–2.45) and for CD was 0.45 (95% CI, 0.24–0.85).[66] In a retrospective study of patients with acne seeking treatment over a 5-year period, the risk of IBD was lower in the isotretinoin-exposed group (unadjusted OR, 0.33; 95% CI, 0.12–0.93; $P = .04$).[67]

Oral antibiotics are associated with IBD based on the results of a meta-analysis of 11 observational studies involving 7208 patients. The overall ORs for antibiotic exposure and CD and UC were 1.74 (95% CI, 1.35–2.23) and 1.08 (95% CI, 0.91–1.27), respectively. In children, an OR for CD was observed of 2.75 (95% CI, 1.72–4.38). All antibiotics, except penicillin, were associated with IBD and highest risks were for metronidazole (OR, 5.01; 95% CI, 1.65–15.25) and fluoroquinolones (OR, 1.79; 95% CI, 1.03–3.12).[68]

Abnormal Wound Healing

Current recommendations to avoid acne scar repair procedures within 6 months after oral isotretinoin arose from reports in the mid-1980s of delayed wound healing and hypertrophic scarring with conventional and argon laser dermabrasion.[69–71] However, recent studies of resurfacing procedures suggest that wound healing is not impaired if treatment is performed earlier. In 10 patients treated within 1 to 3 months after oral isotretinoin with medium-depth peels and manual sandpaper dermabrasion, 6-month follow-up showed no evidence of hypertrophic or keloidal scars.[72,73] In 20 patients treated with ablative carbon dioxide laser within 1 to 3 months after oral isotretinoin, no hypertrophic scars/keloids were noted at 6-month follow-up.[74] An additional study of patients on low-dose isotretinoin (10 mg/d) showed no abnormal scars after nonablative infrared fractional laser.[75]

Recent animal studies have corroborated these findings. In rabbits, 40 wounds created with 6-mm punch biopsies in the ears of 2 control and 2 experimental rabbits (the latter fed isotretinoin 4 mg/kg/d) showed no difference in wound healing clinically or histologically. Collagen synthesis was also similarly unaffected.[76] In minipigs, a model with similarity to human cutaneous structure and wound repair, standard full-thickness (punch biopsies) and partial-thickness (phenol peel) injuries were evaluated over 28 days in an animal treated with isotretinoin (2 mg/kg/d over a 60-day period, attaining a cumulative dose of 120 mg/kg) and a control without treatment. Histologic and photographic measures of wound healing did not differ at 7, 14, or 28 days.[77]

SUMMARY

Over the past decade, progress in basic and clinical research on isotretinoin use in acne has resulted in developments relevant to clinicians involved with acne management. Sebocyte apoptosis and inhibition of TLR-2 levels underlie some of the mechanisms of action of oral isotretinoin in acne leading to sebosuppression and antiinflammatory effects. New evidence suggests that suppression of certain hormones implicated in acne may also be relevant. Variability in bioavailability in individual patients may be caused by different forms of isotretinoin (innovator, isotretinoin-Lidose, and generic formulations), varying fat content of coingestants, and irregular eating habits. There is a trend to higher cumulative doses of isotretinoin required to achieve acne clearance with increasing acne severity when dosed to the clinical end point of no new acne lesions for 1 month. Higher cumulative doses of oral isotretinoin result in greater potential for remission than lower doses. There is no moderate-grade or high-grade evidence supporting the concept of cumulative threshold isotretinoin dosing of 120 to 150 mg/kg. Current studies on relapse are highly flawed by inconsistent and variable definitions of clearance and relapse.

For mitigation of harms, contraception counseling within pregnancy prevention programs should include information on effectiveness of all methods, including long-acting reversible contraception. Adherence to abstinence may be problematic in patients who were previously sexually active. For depression, both acne and isotretinoin may confer a slight increase in risk. Current evidence does not support an association of oral isotretinoin and IBD. However, the association of IBD with systemic antibiotics should be of concern to dermatologists because of their widespread use in treatment of acne and other acneiform dermatoses. Recommendations to avoid acne scar repair procedures within 6 months after using isotretinoin should be reconsidered. Earlier treatment of scarring may provide hope that this issue can be effectively addressed on a timely basis.

REFERENCES

1. Thiboutot D, Gollnick H, Bettoli V, et al. Oral isotretinoin and pregnancy prevention programmes. Br J Dermatol 2012;166(2):466–7.
2. Wolverton SE, Harper JC. Important controversies associated with isotretinoin therapy for acne. Am J Clin Dermatol 2013;14(2):71–6.
3. Goodfield MJ, Cox NH, Bowser A, et al. Advice on the safe introduction and continued use of isotretinoin in acne in the U.K. 2010. Br J Dermatol 2010; 162(6):1172–9.
4. Rowe C, Spelman L, Oziemski M, et al. Isotretinoin and mental health in adolescents: Australian consensus. Australas J Dermatol 2013;55(2):162–7.
5. Zouboulis CC, Bettoli V. Management of severe acne. Br J Dermatol 2015;172(Suppl 1):27–36.
6. On SC, Zeichner J. Isotretinoin updates. Dermatol Ther 2013;26(5):377–89.
7. Layton A. The use of isotretinoin in acne. Dermatoendocrinol 2009;1(3):162–9.
8. Nelson AM, Gilliland KL, Cong Z, et al. 13-cis retinoic acid induces apoptosis and cell cycle arrest in human SEB-1 sebocytes. J Invest Dermatol 2006; 126(10):2178–89.
9. Nelson AM, Cong Z, Gilliland KL, et al. TRAIL contributes to the apoptotic effect of 13-cis retinoic acid in human sebaceous gland cells. Br J Dermatol 2011;165(3):526–33.
10. Nelson AM, Zhao W, Gilliland KL, et al. Neutrophil gelatinase–associated lipocalin mediates 13-cis retinoic acid–induced apoptosis of human sebaceous gland cells. J Clin Invest 2008;118(4):1468–78.
11. Lumsden KR, Nelson AM, Dispenza MC, et al. Isotretinoin increases skin-surface levels of neutrophil gelatinase-associated lipocalin in patients treated for severe acne. Br J Dermatol 2011; 165(2):302–10.
12. Dispenza MC, Wolpert EB, Gilliland KL, et al. Systemic isotretinoin therapy normalizes exaggerated TLR-2-mediated innate immune responses in acne patients. J Invest Dermatol 2012;132(9):2198–205.
13. Karadag AS, Takci Z, Ertugrul DT, et al. The effect of different doses of isotretinoin on pituitary hormones. Dermatology 2015;230:354–9.
14. US Department of Health and Human Services, Food and Drug Administration, Centre for Drug Evaluation and Research (CDER). Guidance for industry: food-effect bioavailability and fed bioequivalence studies. 2002:1–12. Available at: http://www.fda.gov/downloads/RegulatoryInformation/Guidances/UCM126833.pdf.
15. Colburn WA, Gibson DM, Wiens RE, et al. Food increases the bioavailability of isotretinoin. J Clin Pharmacol 1983;23(11–12):534–9.
16. Deshmukh-Taskar PR, Nicklas TA, O'Neil CE, et al. The relationship of breakfast skipping and type of breakfast consumption with nutrient intake and weight status in children and adolescents: the National Health and Nutrition Examination Survey 1999-2006. J Am Diet Assoc 2010;110(6):869–78.
17. Leyden JJ, Del Rosso JQ, Baum EW. The use of isotretinoin in the treatment of acne vulgaris: clinical considerations and future directions. J Clin Aesthet Dermatol 2014;7(2 Suppl):S3–21.
18. Mutizwa MM, Sheinbein DM. Are we underdosing acne patients with generic isotretinoin? Dermatol Online J 2013;19(1):12.
19. Webster GF, Leyden JJ, Gross JA. Results of a phase III, double-blind, randomized, parallel-group, non-inferiority study evaluating the safety and efficacy of isotretinoin-Lidose in patients with severe recalcitrant nodular acne. J Drugs Dermatol 2014;13(6):665–70.
20. Tan J, Humphrey S, Vender R, et al. A treatment for severe nodular acne: a randomized investigator-blinded,

controlled, noninferiority trial comparing fixed-dose adapalene/benzoyl peroxide plus doxycycline vs. oral isotretinoin. Br J Dermatol 2014;171(6):1508–16.

21. Cyrulnik AA, Viola KV, Gewirtzman AJ, et al. High-dose isotretinoin in acne vulgaris: improved treatment outcomes and quality of life. Int J Dermatol 2012;51(9):1123–30.

22. Blasiak RC, Stamey CR, Burkhart CN, et al. High-dose isotretinoin treatment and the rate of retrial, relapse, and adverse effects in patients with acne vulgaris. JAMA Dermatol 2013;149(12):1392–8.

23. Lee JW, Yoo KH, Park KY, et al. Effectiveness of conventional, low-dose and intermittent oral isotretinoin in the treatment of acne: a randomized, controlled comparative study. Br J Dermatol 2011; 164(6):1369–75.

24. Rademaker M. Isotretinoin: dose, duration and relapse. What does 30 years of usage tell us? Australas J Dermatol 2012;54(3):157–62.

25. Sardana K, Garg VK. Low-dose isotretinoin in acne vulgaris: a critical review. Br J Dermatol 2011; 165(3):698–700.

26. Rademaker M. Adverse effects of isotretinoin: a retrospective review of 1743 patients started on isotretinoin. Australas J Dermatol 2010;51(4):248–53.

27. Berk DR. On isotretinoin dosing, adverse effects, and efficacy. Australas J Dermatol 2011;52(2):147–8 [author reply: 148].

28. Borghi A, Mantovani L, Minghetti S, et al. Low-cumulative dose isotretinoin treatment in mild-to-moderate acne: efficacy in achieving stable remission. J Eur Acad Dermatol Venereol 2011;25(9):1094–8.

29. Rademaker M, Wishart JM, Birchall NM. Isotretinoin 5 mg daily for low-grade adult acne vulgaris - a placebo-controlled, randomized double-blind study. J Eur Acad Dermatol Venereol 2014;28(6):747–54.

30. Layton AM, Cunliffe WJ. Guidelines for optimal use of isotretinoin in acne. J Am Acad Dermatol 1992; 27(6 Pt 2):S2–7.

31. Cunliffe WJ, van de Kerkhof PC, Caputo R, et al. Roaccutane treatment guidelines: results of an international survey. Dermatology 1997;194(4):351–7.

32. Zeichner J. On Dosage and Diet: Isotretinoin 101. Pract Dermatol 2014;46–7.

33. Del Rosso JQ. Face to face with oral isotretinoin: a closer look at the spectrum of therapeutic outcomes and why some patients need repeated courses. J Clin Aesthet Dermatol 2012;5(11):17–24.

34. Strauss JS, Krowchuk DP, Leyden JJ, et al. Guidelines of care for acne vulgaris management. J Am Acad Dermatol 2007;56(4):651–63.

35. Malaysia Ministry of Health, Dermatological Society of Malaysia, Academy of Medicine Malaysia. Clinical practice guidelines: management of acne. 2012. Available at: http://www.moh.gov.my. Accessed July 15, 2012.

36. Nast A, Dreno B, Bettoli V, et al. European evidence-based (S3) guidelines for the treatment of acne. J Eur Acad Dermatol Venereol 2012;26:1–29.

37. Azoulay L, Oraichi D, Bérard A. Isotretinoin therapy and the incidence of acne relapse: a nested case-control study. Br J Dermatol 2007;157(6):1240–8.

38. Tan JLK, Knezevic S, Boyal S, et al. Evaluation of evidence for acne remission with oral isotretinoin cumulative dosing of 120-150 mg/kg. J Cutan Med Surg 2015. [Epub ahead of print].

39. Yook JH, Han JY, Choi JS, et al. Pregnancy outcomes and factors associated with voluntary pregnancy termination in women who had been treated for acne with isotretinoin. Clin Toxicol 2012;50(10):896–901.

40. Zomerdijk IM, Ruiter R, Houweling LM, et al. Isotretinoin exposure during pregnancy: a population-based study in The Netherlands. BMJ Open 2014; 4(11):e005602.

41. Pinheiro SP, Kang EM, Kim CY, et al. Concomitant use of isotretinoin and contraceptives before and after iPledge in the United States. Pharmacoepidemiol Drug Saf 2013;22(12):1251–7.

42. Collins MK, Moreau JF, Opel D, et al. Compliance with pregnancy prevention measures during isotretinoin therapy. J Am Acad Dermatol 2014;70(1):55–9.

43. Werner CA, Papic MJ, Ferris LK, et al. Women's experiences with isotretinoin risk reduction counseling. JAMA Dermatol 2014;150(4):366–71.

44. Lam C, Zaenglein AL. Contraceptive use in acne. Clin Dermatol 2014;32(4):502–15.

45. Thiboutot D, Zaenglein A. Isotretinoin and affective disorders: thirty years later. J Am Acad Dermatol 2013;68(4):675–6.

46. Kontaxakis VP, Skourides D, Ferentinos P, et al. Isotretinoin and psychopathology: a review. Ann Gen Psychiatry 2009;8:2.

47. Misery L. Consequences of psychological distress in adolescents with acne. J Invest Dermatol 2010; 131(2):290–2.

48. Borovaya A, Olisova O, Ruzicka T, et al. Does isotretinoin therapy of acne cure or cause depression? Int J Dermatol 2013;52(9):1040–52.

49. D'Erme AM, Pinelli S, Cossidente A, et al. Association between isotretinoin and mood changes: myth or reality? An updated overview. Int J Dermatol 2011;52(4):499–500.

50. Bremner JD, Shearer K, McCaffery P. Retinoic acid and affective disorders: the evidence for an association. J Clin Psychiatry 2012;73:37–50.

51. Strauss JS, Leyden JJ, Lucky AW, et al. Safety of a new micronized formulation of isotretinoin in patients with severe recalcitrant nodular acne: a randomized trial comparing micronized isotretinoin with standard isotretinoin. J Am Acad Dermatol 2001;45(2):196–207.

52. Scheinman PL, Peck GL, Rubinow DR, et al. Acute depression from isotretinoin. J Am Acad Dermatol 1990;22:1112–4.

53. Azoulay L, Blais L, Koren G, et al. Isotretinoin and the risk of depression in patients with acne vulgaris: a case-crossover study. J Clin Psychiatry 2008;69: 526–32.

54. Lewinsohn PM, Hops H, Roberts RE, et al. Adolescent psychopathology: I. Prevalence and incidence of depression and other DSM-III-R disorders in high school students. J Abnorm Psychol 1993;102: 133–44.

55. Halvorsen JA, Stern RS, Dalgard F, et al. Suicidal ideation, mental health problems, and social impairment are increased in adolescents with acne: a population-based study. J Invest Dermatol 2011; 131(2):363–70.

56. Sundström A, Alfredsson L, Sjölin-Forsberg G, et al. Association of suicide attempts with acne and treatment with isotretinoin: retrospective Swedish cohort study. BMJ 2010;341:c5812.

57. Löwe B, Kroenke K, Gräfe K. Detecting and monitoring depression with a two-item questionnaire (PHQ-2). J Psychosom Res 2005;58(2):163–71.

58. Kroenke K, Spitzer RL, Williams JB. The patient health questionnaire-2: validity of a two-item depression screener. Med Care 2003;41(11):1284–92.

59. Gilbody S, Richards D, Brealey S, et al. Screening for depression in medical settings with the Patient Health Questionnaire (PHQ): a diagnostic meta-analysis. J Gen Intern Med 2007;22(11):1596–602.

60. Bagby RM, Ryder AG, Schuller DR, et al. The Hamilton Depression Rating Scale: has the gold standard become a lead weight? Am J Psychiatry 2004; 161(12):2163–77.

61. Ebell MH. Screening instruments for depression. Am Fam Physician 2008;78(2):244–6.

62. Bernstein CN, Nugent Z, Longobardi T, et al. Isotretinoin is not associated with inflammatory bowel disease: a population-based case-control study. Am J Gastroenterol 2009;104(11):2774–8.

63. Crockett SD, Porter CQ, Martin CF, et al. Isotretinoin use and the risk of inflammatory bowel disease: a case-control study. Am J Gastroenterol 2010;105: 1986–93.

64. Etminan M, Bird ST, Delaney JA, et al. Isotretinoin and risk for inflammatory bowel disease: a nested case-control study and meta-analysis of published and unpublished data. JAMA Dermatol 2013; 149(2):216–20.

65. Alhusayen RO, Juurlink DN, Mamdani MM, et al. Isotretinoin use and the risk of inflammatory bowel disease: a population-based cohort study. J Invest Dermatol 2013;133(4):907–12.

66. Racine A, Cuerq A, Bijon A, et al. Isotretinoin and risk of inflammatory bowel disease: a French nationwide study. Am J Gastroenterol 2014;109(4):563–9.

67. Rashtak S, Khaleghi S, Pittelkow MR, et al. Isotretinoin exposure and risk of inflammatory bowel disease. JAMA Dermatol 2014;150(12):1322–6.

68. Ungaro R, Bernstein CN, Gearry R, et al. Antibiotics associated with increased risk of new-onset Crohn's disease but not ulcerative colitis: a meta-analysis. Am J Gastroenterol 2014;109(11):1728–38.

69. Rubenstein R, Roenigk HH Jr, Stegman SJ, et al. Atypical keloids after dermabrasion of patients taking isotretinoin. J Am Acad Dermatol 1986;15(2 Pt 1):280–5.

70. Katz BE, Mac Farlane DF. Atypical facial scarring after isotretinoin therapy in a patient with previous dermabrasion. J Am Acad Dermatol 1994;30(5 Pt 2):852–3.

71. Zachariae H. Delayed wound healing and keloid formation following argon laser treatment or dermabrasion during isotretinoin treatment. Br J Dermatol 1988;118(5):703–6.

72. Picosse FR, Yarak S, Cabral NC, et al. Early chemabrasion for acne scars after treatment with oral isotretinoin. Dermatol Surg 2012;38(9):1521–6.

73. Bagatin E, dos Santos Guadanhim LR, Yarak S, et al. Dermabrasion for acne scars during treatment with oral isotretinoin. Dermatol Surg 2010;36(4):483–9.

74. Kim HW, Chang SE, Kim JE, et al. The safe delivery of fractional ablative carbon dioxide laser treatment for acne scars in Asian patients receiving oral isotretinoin. Dermatol Surg 2014;40(12):1361–6.

75. Yoon JH, Park EJ, Kwon IH, et al. Concomitant use of an infrared fractional laser with low-dose isotretinoin for the treatment of acne and acne scars. J Dermatolog Treat 2014;25(2):142–6.

76. Moy RL, Moy LS, Bennett RG, et al. Systemic isotretinoin: effects on dermal wound healing in a rabbit ear model in vivo. J Dermatol Surg Oncol 1990;16: 1142–6.

77. Larson DL, Flugstad NA, O'Connor E, et al. Does systemic isotretinoin inhibit healing in a porcine wound model? Aesthet Surg J 2012;32(8):989–98.

Safety Considerations and Monitoring in Patients Treated with Systemic Medications for Acne

CrossMark

Hyunhee Park, DO[a],*, Stanley Skopit, DO, MSE[b]

KEYWORDS

• Acne • Systemic treatments • Safety • Monitoring • Oral antibiotics • Spironolactone • Isotretinoin

KEY POINTS

• Minocycline-induced autoimmunity and hypersensitivity reactions have been increasingly reported in the last few decades.
• Doxycycline is rarely associated with serious adverse effects over more recent years.
• There is literature to support that routine monitoring of serum potassium levels in healthy young women taking spironolactone for acne is not necessary.
• Ocular adverse effects of isotretinoin may need to be communicated to the patients more actively for better safety monitoring.
• Low-dose intermittent isotretinoin regimen has been reported effective.

INTRODUCTION

Acne vulgaris is one of the most commonly encountered conditions in dermatology practice. It is a disorder of the pilosebaceous unit and affects about 33% of individuals between the ages 15 and 44 years, primarily adolescents.[1] Effective treatment of acne vulgaris is important in that it can prevent psychosocial distress and physical scarring. Various therapeutic options are available according to the severity of the disease. Although a broad proportion of patients with acne can be successfully treated using topical agents such as benzoyl peroxide, topical antibiotics, and topical retinoids, patients with moderate to severe inflammatory acne require systemic therapy. This article is a concise review of side effects and monitoring guide for the most commonly prescribed systemic agents for acne vulgaris.

TETRACYCLINES

Tetracyclines are the most commonly prescribed antibiotics for the treatment of acne. Compared with the original tetracycline, the second-generation synthetic molecules, doxycycline and minocycline, offer easier dosing schedules and are more readily absorbed when taken with food.[2] They are bacteriostatic and work on inhibition of bacterial protein synthesis. Serious side effects associated with tetracyclines are rare in its use for acne, but as an antibiotic class, more common side effects of doxycycline and minocycline include gastrointestinal symptoms with nausea, vomiting, and diarrhea; pediatric teeth discoloration; central nervous system effects such as dizziness and light headedness; and candidiasis.[2,3] Photosensitivity and photo-onycholysis are also seen,[4] however, sun protection with daily

[a] Department of Dermatology, Larkin Community Hospital/NSU-COM, 4970 West Atlantic Boulevard, Margate, FL 33063, USA; [b] Dermatology Residency Program, Larkin Community Hospital/NSU-COM, 4970 West Atlantic Boulevard, Margate, FL 33063, USA
* Corresponding author.
E-mail address: hparkdo@gmail.com

Dermatol Clin 34 (2016) 185–193
http://dx.doi.org/10.1016/j.det.2015.11.004
0733-8635/16/$ – see front matter © 2016 Elsevier Inc. All rights reserved.

sunscreen wear may help prevent treatment-related sunburns. Doxycycline and minocycline offer similar efficacy for management of acne,[5–7] but they differ in their side-effect profiles. Recent literature reviews have compared the safety profiles of doxycycline and minocycline.[2,3]

In their systematic review of safety of doxycycline and minocycline, Smith and and Leyden noted that there were more than 3 times as many new prescriptions for doxycycline than for minocycline in the United States from 1998 to 2003. And the adverse event rates for the same period were 5 times greater for minocycline than doxycycline based on the US Food and Drug Administration's MedWatch Adverse Event reporting program data. Analysis by Smith and Leyden[2] also found that gastrointestinal effects were the most common adverse effects related to doxycycline use, whereas central nervous system and gastrointestinal effects were most common with minocycline. In this 2005 article, Smith and Leyden[2] made an observation regarding the kinds of adverse effects that differed from clinical trials and published case reports. For doxycycline, the types of adverse effects in published case reports were similar to those reported in clinical trials. However, those for minocycline were significantly different, with events that range from minocycline-induced drug reaction with eosinophilia and systemic symptoms (DRESS) syndrome with persistent myocarditis to minocycline-induced autoimmunity (MIA).[8,9] The authors noted that case reports represent something of clinical interest to the medical community and generally reflect less frequent but more serious adverse effects. However, taken collectively, the patterns of reported adverse events can suggest a causal relationship between the drug and event, justifying further investigation.[2]

According to Kircik[3] in his 2010 article, data indicate that MIA may lead to chronic symptoms, persisting from 13 to 48 months.[10] Pathogenesis of MIA has not yet been established, although it is suspected to be similar to other drug-induced autoimmunity.[3] Female patients are more commonly affected than male patients. The average age of onset of MIA was between 13 and 18 years with mean duration of minocycline therapy of 13 months for those with transient MIA, 14.6 months for those with intermediate, and 11.8 for those with chronic MIA. The median estimated cumulative minocycline dose in each of the 3 groups was 72 g, and most patients had a positive family history of autoimmune disorder.[10]

Minocycline is also associated with potentially fatal hypersensitivity syndrome or DRESS.[8,11] Predictive factors are not well defined, but recent evidence suggests that minocycline-induced

DRESS occurs mainly in patients with Fitzpatrick skin phototypes V and VI.[12] Although the incidence of minocycline-induced DRESS is rare, its widespread use necessitates awareness among physicians who are initiating systemic antiacne therapy in patients, especially those with skin types V and VI.

Doxycycline, however is viewed as the safest within the tetracycline class, with fewer reported cases of side effects.[13] It is available in 2 different formulations: doxycycline hyclate and doxycycline monohydrate. Doxycycline hyclate is more acidic than doxycycline monohydrate and may be associated with a higher risk of esophageal ulceration if the drug is taken without sufficient water.[3] The development of enteric-coated doxycycline hyclate has been linked to a decrease in gastrointestinal side effects.[14] Also, taking it with adequate amount of water is found to significantly decrease the risk of esophageal ulceration.[4] Studies support the benefit of enteric-coated doxycycline to decrease nausea, vomiting, and abdominal pain compared with both conventional doxycycline hyclate capsule and doxycycline monohydrate.[15,16] Despite its favorable safety record, several serious doxycycline-induced adverse reactions have emerged over the last few years.[17] There are several case reports of doxycycline-induced pseudotumor cerebri in acne patients and DRESS syndrome after doxycycline treatment.[18–21] One case of doxycycline-induced cutaneous inflammation with systemic symptoms was also reported in a 15-year-old patient taking doxycycline for 2 years.[17] A brief summary of adverse reactions to minocycline and doxycycline is outlined in **Table 1**.

SPIRONOLACTONE

Although not approved by the US Food and Drug Administration for the treatment of acne, spironolactone, a medicine that blocks androgen receptors, is found to be effective in treating acne vulgaris, at daily dosage of 100 to 200 mg, in most women and adolescent girls, especially those with worsening acne associated with menstrual cycle.[31–34] The incidence of side effects at this dose may be high, ranging from 75% to 91%, but the severity is generally mild with good tolerance by most women.[35] Reported side effects included menstrual irregularities and central nervous system side effects such as headache and dizziness.[36] More recent data support the efficacy of lower doses of spironolactone at 50 to 100 mg daily, which were much better tolerated.[31,35,37,38] The main side effect reported at this dose was mild, clinically insignificant elevation of serum

Table 1
Adverse reactions associated with minocycline and doxycycline

Antibiotic	Adverse Reaction	Studies
Minocycline	Vomiting/abdominal pain/diarrhea	Smith & Leyden,[2] Kircik[3]
	Vertigo/dizziness/light headedness/ataxia	Smith & Leyden,[2] Kircik,[3] Meynadier & Alirezai[22]
	Candidiasis	Smith & Leyden,[2] Kircik[3]
	Photosensitivity/photo-onycholysis	Sloan & Scheinfeld[4]
	Bluish discoloration of the skin	Tan[23]
	DRESS	Shaughnessy et al,[8] Eshki et al,[11] Maubec et al[12]
	MIA—lupus, autoimmune hepatitis, serum sickness, vasculitis	Elkayam et al,[9] El-Hallak et al,[10] Matsuura et al,[24] Sturkenboom et al,[25] Schlienger et al,[26] Seaman et al[27]
	Pneumonitis	Christodoulou et al[28]
Doxycycline	Vomiting/abdominal pain/diarrhea	Smith & Leyden,[2] Kircik,[3] Story et al,[15] Jarvinen[16]
	Dizziness/light headedness	Smith & Leyden,[2] Kircik[3]
	Candidiasis	Smith & Leyden,[2] Kircik[3]
	Photosensitivity/photo-onycholysis	Sloan & Scheinfeld,[4] Edwards[29]
	Acute generalized exanthematous pustulosis	Trueb & Burg[30]
	Esophageal ulceration	Kircik,[3] Sloan & Scheinfeld,[4] Berger[14]
	Pseudotumor cerebri	Tabibian & Gutierrez,[18] Friedman et al[19]
	DRESS (data very limited)	Robles et al,[20] Mailhol et al[21]
	Cutaneous inflammation with systemic symptoms (15 y-old patient taking doxycycline daily for 2 y)	Weinstein et al[17]

potassium levels.[39] Plovanich and colleagues most recently report the results on the monitoring of serum potassium level for this potential hyperkalemia among healthy young women taking spironolactone for acne in their electronically published article in March 2015. Based on their data from a retrospective study of 974 healthy young women taking spironolactone from 2000 to 2014, they noted 13 abnormal serum potassium measurements in 1802 measurements obtained. This finding yielded a rate of 0.72% for hyperkalemia compared with 0.76% baseline rate of hyperkalemia in this population. Furthermore, the repeat testing in 6 of 13 patients found normal values, suggesting that the findings might have been erroneous. Considering this new establishment of hyperkalemia incidence, which is equivalent to the baseline rate in this population, Plovanich and colleagues[40] concluded that routine potassium monitoring is unnecessary in healthy young women taking spironolactone for acne. A list of reported adverse reactions associated with spironolactone is outlined in **Table 2**.

ISOTRETINOIN

The clinical adverse effects of isotretinoin can be grouped into 2 categories: mucocutaneous and systemic. Of the adverse effects reported, those that occur with highest incidence are mucocutaneous in nature and usually noticeable within the first week of therapy. This effect is caused by

Table 2
Adverse reactions associated with Spironolactone

Reaction Pattern	Studies
Menstrual irregularities	Shaw,[31] Shaw,[35] Hughes & Cunliffe,[36] Shaw,[37] Yemisci et al,[38] Lubbos et al[41]
Breast tenderness or enlargement	Shaw,[37] Cunliffe & Simpson[42]
Headache	Shaw,[37] Lubbos et al[41]
Fatigue	Shaw,[31] Shaw[37]
Dizziness	Shaw,[35] Yemisci et al[38]
Drowsiness	Shaw[35]
Nausea/vomiting/diarrhea/anorexia	Shaw,[35] Shaw[38]
Decreased libido	Shaw[35]
Hyperkalemia	Shaw,[37] Plovanich et al[40]
Melasma	Shaw[37]
Facial swelling	Lubbos et al[41]

changes in mucosal surfaces and skin that have been altered in the barrier function from the reduction in sebum production leading to thinning of the stratum corneum.[43–45]

Most patients have dryness and fissures on the lips, skin, and mucosa. Lip dryness occurs in 100% of the cases and cheilitis in 95% of the cases.[43,46] This dose-related cheilitis is so common that some elucidate it is a marker of the action of the isotretinoin.[47] On the other hand, complete absence of cheilitis may suggest noncompliance or malabsorption of the drug.[45] Dryness of the nasal and oral mucosa have been reported in 50% and 40%, respectively.[46] Dry eyes and blepharoconjunctivitis develop in 25% of the patients and are controlled with eye lubricants.[46]

The ocular side effects tend to be less emphasized despite their frequent report along with lip dryness. Neudorfer and colleagues[48] looked at the study population of 14,682 adolescents and young adults who were new users of isotretinoin for acne and 2 age- and sex-matched comparison groups. They described the most common adverse effects and evaluated the period of highest risk. The most common adverse effects in Neudorfer's study included conjunctivitis, hordeolum, chalazion, blepharitis, eye pain, and dry eye, which is in agreement with findings from previous studies.[48,49] Development of these ocular adverse effects took place with the peak increased risk at 4 months after the first dispensed isotretinoin prescription, advocating for a follow-up visit to the ophthalmologist around that time.[48] The results of this study underscore the importance of proper prevention and management measures and the most optimal timeframe to detect any significant ocular adverse effects. Ocular lubricants such as preservative-free artificial tears can be prescribed, but in more severe cases, topical ophthalmologic antibiotics may be needed. The health care provider must be aware of these potential side effects when educating patients, because some events are reported to be irreversible, even during periods of acute exposure to isotretinoin.[48,50,51]

In 2010, Brito and colleagues[43] published a study in which they evaluated the clinical adverse effects and laboratory alterations in patients with acne treated with oral isotretinoin. Of the 150 patients, the frequency of the mucocutaneous adverse effects was similar to that found in the literature. Cheilitis (94%) was the most common followed by xeroderma and dryness of mucous membranes (47%). Despite this high rate of mucocutaneous effects, symptoms were managed with lip balm and body moisturizers, eye drops, and ophthalmologic evaluation, and none of the effects served as a reason to suspend the drug in Brito's study. They also noted the incident of pyogenic granuloma in 13% of the cases but without any case resulting in the suspension of isotretinoin.[43] There was a report of 3 cases of granulomalike reactions in 66 patients (4.5%) treated with isotretinoin for nodulocystic acne. Pyogenic granulomalike reactions developed in previous acne lesions and led to discontinuation of the drug in 2 of them. The exact incidence of pyogenic granuloma or granulomalike reactions secondary to the use of isotretinoin is unknown.[43,52]

Mucocutaneous effects usually persist throughout the treatment course but have been documented to be reversible at the time of dosage reduction or discontinuation of the drug.[53] Most of these effects can be efficiently managed through the use of mild soaps, facial washing limited to once a day, avoidance of concurrent use of other acne medications, use of hydrating moisturizers, use of sunscreen, and frequent lip lubrication with a petroleum product.[51,54] Patients should be instructed to avoid cosmetic procedures such as dermabrasion, waxing, and laser treatment for up to 6 months after isotretinoin therapy because of complications including potential keloid formation and delayed wound healing.[55–57]

The systemic toxicity of retinoid may affect bones, muscles, gastrointestinal tract, central nervous system, lungs, ears, and kidneys. Isotretinoin use by patients with acne usually does not cause serious bone changes. Although hyperostosis are considered irreversible,[58] they are generally asymptomatic and insignificant even with long-term use.[59] In addition to hyperostosis, case reports of premature epiphyseal closures have been described with high doses of isotretinoin, but it may be reversible.[55,60] Myalgia can occur, especially in patients who exhibit vigorous physical activity. In general, however, elevation in creatine phosphokinase level is relatively uncommon and usually reversible.[61,62] Myalgia can usually be controlled with nonsteroidal anti-inflammatory drugs. Adverse gastrointestinal effects related to isotretinoin therapy seem to be reversible after therapy cessation[63] and range from nausea and other nonspecific gastrointestinal effects to pancreatitis, hepatitis, appendicitis, esophagitis, and colitis.[55,64,65] There are conflicting reports regarding the possibility of isotretinoin causing or exacerbating the symptoms of inflammatory bowel disease[55,66,67]; however history of inflammatory bowel disease does not seem to be an absolute contraindication for isotretinoin use for nodulocystic or recalcitrant acne among current practitioners. Neurologic reactions reported to occur with isotretinoin use are rare. They include idiopathic increases in intracranial pressure, confusion, dizziness, drowsiness, seizures, lethargy, malaise, nervousness, syncope, weakness, paresthesias, stroke, and pseudotumor cerebri presenting with headache, nausea, vomiting, and visual disturbances.[44,51,68–70] Such symptoms should be carefully discussed, and a referral to a neurologist may be warranted. Despite the adverse pulmonary effects associated with isotretinoin therapy, specific pulmonary events such as bronchospasm and asthma exacerbation have been noted.[71,72] Monitoring of the pulmonary function may be required in individuals with this response for proper reduction of dose or termination of therapy. Among other uncommon events that are reported in the literature, hearing impairment is significant to recognize, as it does not disappear after the suspension of isotretinoin.[73] The mechanism that causes this deterioration in hearing is unknown, and patients must be evaluated by otorhinolaryngologist. Besides hearing impairment, tinnitus has also been described.[73] Other nonspecific hearing problems were identified by Brito and colleagues[43] in 2010, which did not lead to suspension of the drug. Adverse renal effects related to isotretinoin use are rare, with a few cases of glomerulonephritis, urethritis, and proteinuria.[74,75] These renal abnormalities resolve after discontinuation of isotretinoin therapy.[74]

With regard to psychiatric effects attributed to isotretinoin, controversies exist over a causal relationship between treatment with isotretinoin and psychiatric symptoms with the reports of depression, psychoses, suicidal thoughts, and suicide attempts.[76,77] However, there are doubts about this association.[78–80] A 2001 cohort study conducted in Canada looked at 7535 patients treated with isotretinoin and 14,376 patients treated with oral antibiotics. The study compared the relative estimated risk of suicide among patients with acne treated with isotretinoin or oral antibiotics, but an association between isotretinoin use and an increased risk of suicide was not found.[79] Physicians' concerns for the psychiatric adverse effects have not subsided, and continuing efforts with educating patients, especially those with a history of depression, to immediately report changes in moods or behavior, suicidal thoughts, or feelings need to be regularly practiced.

Among the adverse side effects of isotretinoin, teratogenicity is considered the most serious. Specific teratogenic effects involve craniofacial, cardiac, thymic, and central nervous system structures.[68,81,82] These findings have resulted in a stringent management of the medication with birth control policy, which includes 2 pregnancy tests before initiation of therapy, 2 forms of

contraception to be used throughout the therapy, contraception education, and the required informed consent for patients.[81] All patients should re-review the information in the informed consent form at each monthly follow-up visit. It is imperative that only 1-month supply of isotretinoin be prescribed at any office visit after documentation of the absence of pregnancy. Patients must be counseled that pregnancy prevention should continue 1 month after discontinuation of therapy. It is a standard practice at some dermatologists' offices to formulate these into a checklist and use as protocol for initial and follow-up appointments.[51]

In addition to monthly pregnancy testing, review of any laboratory alterations are necessary before continuing isotretinoin therapy. Of the laboratory abnormalities, liver functions tests and lipid abnormalities are most critical to assess. Despite the fact that 5% to 25% of patients treated with isotretinoin show some abnormalities in the liver function tests, most of these cases are without any histologic liver changes, and the elevated levels of hepatic enzymes return to normal after discontinuing isotretinoin therapy or with dose reduction.[55,83] As a general rule, dose reduction should be considered when the liver function results are 2- to 3-fold their normal value, and if they do not decrease with dose reduction after 2 weeks, discontinuation of isotretinoin may be necessary. Elevations of transaminase levels greater than 3 times the upper normal value warrant immediate cessation of therapy.[84] Monitoring of liver function is especially critical in patients with underlying liver disease or history of hepatitis. It is recommended that health care providers also educate patients on the concomitant use of hepatotoxins, such as alcohol and other drugs, which may contribute to hepatic function test abnormalities. Evaluation of liver function tests at baseline before isotretinoin therapy and at follow-up appointment at each month is a standard safety practice in this regard. Lipid abnormalities are another well-documented adverse effect of isotretinoin therapy requiring a sound monitoring. These effects include decreased serum levels of high-density lipoprotein cholesterol, increased serum levels of very low-density lipoprotein cholesterol and low-density lipoprotein cholesterol, and increased serum total cholesterol levels.[85] Increased triglyceride levels are seen in 25% to 45% of patients on isotretinoin.[86] Although significant variations of serum lipid and lipoprotein levels do not affect the overall risk of atherosclerosis in young and healthy patients on short courses of isotretinoin, continuous isotretinoin use in patients with underlying lipid disorders may lead to an increased risk of cardiovascular event.[51,86] Although rare, cases of isotretinoin-induced pancreatitis secondary to hypertriglyceridemia have also been reported.[55] For this reason, if pancreatitis is suspected, or if hyperlipidemia is not controlled with antihyperlipidemic medicines, it is important to suspend isotretinoin use.[55,87] In general, dose reduction or the introduction of antihyperlipidemic agent is considered when triglyceride level exceeds 500 to 600 mg/dL in an otherwise asymptomatic patient.[84] Other reversible and dose-dependent laboratory abnormalities reported in the literature are decreased white blood cell and neutrophil counts, increased platelet counts, thrombocytopenia, and increased erythrocyte sedimentation rates.[51,86,88]

Other adverse effects that are less common but worthwhile to note are photosensitivity, pruritus, hair loss, and skin infections. Photosensitivity appears in 40% of the cases.[43] Pruritus, scaly skin, and worsening of atopic dermatitis occur in 25%.[46] Telogen effluvium may be found in up to 25% of the patients, resolving after discontinuation of the isotretinoin treatment.[43] Skin infections caused by Staphylococcus aureus may develop because of an increase in its colonization resulting from a reduction in sebum production.[46,89]

The aforementioned use of oral isotretinoin in conventional dose administration has been limited by its reported side effects including mucocutaneous adverse effects, teratogenicity, depression with suicidal ideation, and biochemical abnormalities, such as impaired liver function and hyperlipidemia.[90] The low-dose intermittent isotretinoin regimen was devised as a low-cost alternative to the conventional dose regimen, also in effort to reduce the occurrences of adverse effects of isotretinoin.[91] The low-dose intermittent regimen consists of isotretinoin, 0.5 mg/kg/d for 1 week in every 4 weeks for a total period of 6 months. The efficacy of this regimen for mild to severe acne has been established by different studies.[92,93] Various fixed low-dose isotretinoin regimens have also been emerged, and one such regimen with fixed low-dose isotretinoin, 20 mg/d and 20 mg on alternate days for a total period of 6 months, is found to be effective in moderate acne.[94,95] Previous data exist to support that the frequency and severity of mucocutaneous side effects were lower with this low-dose intermittent regimen than with conventional isotretinoin therapy.[93] In an uncontrolled, open-label observational study, Kumar and Kumar[96] evaluated hematologic, biochemical, and radiologic abnormalities associated with low-dose intermittent isotretinoin therapy at 0.5 mg/kg/d for 1 week every 4 weeks for a duration of 6 months. In their study,

liver function results, including total bilirubin levels and transaminase levels, remained within normal limits in all cases. Increase in cholesterol to borderline-high levels (200–239 mg/dL) was observed in 8.3% cases, whereas increase to high levels (≥240 mg/dL) was observed in only 5% of cases after low-dose intermittent isotretinoin.[96] Compared with 30% elevation in cholesterol levels after conventional dose of isotretinoin, the results added to the safety data of low-dose intermittent isotretinoin therapy favorably.[90] Elevation in triglycerides and low-density lipoprotein levels revealed similar outcomes. Furthermore, neither the radiologic changes consistent with diffuse interskeletal hyperostosis of the spine nor the hematologic changes such as leukopenia and increased platelet counts were observed in any case in the Kumar study.[96]

Throughout the last 20 years, the frequency of rigorous laboratory monitoring has decreased, and some of the recent studies show that there is no need for laboratory follow-up in patients taking isotretinoin.[43,97–101] Although there remains a resistance to the use of isotretinoin, especially for milder cases of acne that are irresponsive to conventional therapies, isotretinoin can now be viewed as a reasonably safe drug in relation to adverse effects when the patient is well monitored.[43]

SUMMARY

Systemic therapeutic options are available for moderate to severe acne. It is imperative that the safe and effective treatment revolves around the health care provider's familiarity of side effects of various treatments. When health care providers are equipped with knowledge of various adverse effects of acne treatment, more desirable choices can be made confidently about which treatment options are most appropriate for a particular patient. Moreover, patient education on the possible adverse effects of the prescribed medications can be beneficial in monitoring, with constant vigilance and screening for the development of side effects regardless of the length of treatment.

REFERENCES

1. Stern RS. The prevalence of acne on the basis of physical examination. J Am Acad Dermatol 1992; 26:931–5.
2. Smith K, Leyden JJ. Safety of doxycycline and minocycline: a systemic review. Clin Ther 2005;27(9): 1329–42.
3. Kircik LH. Doxycycline and minocycline for the management of acne: a review of efficacy and

safety with emphasis on clinical implications. J Drugs Dermatol 2010;9(11):1407–11.

4. Sloan B, Scheinfeld N. The use and safety of doxycycline hyclate and other second generation tetracyclines. Expert Opin Drug Saf 2008; 7:571–7.

5. Smit F. Minocycline versus doxycycline in the treatment of acne vulgaris: a double-blind study. Dermatologica 1978;157(3):186–90.

6. Olafsson JH, Gudgerisson J, Eggertsdottir GE, et al. Doxycycline versus minocycline in the treatment of acne vulgaris: a double-blind study. J Dermatolog Treat 1989;1:15–7.

7. Harrison PV. A comparison of doxycycline and minocycline in the treatment of acne vulgaris. Clin Exp Dermatol 1988;13:242–4.

8. Shaughnessy KK, Bouchard SM, Mohr MR, et al. Minocycline-induced drug reaction with eosinophilia and systemic symptoms (DRESS) syndrome with persistent myocarditis. J Am Acad Dermatol 2010;62:315–8.

9. Elkayam O, Yaron M, Caspi D. Minocycline-induced autoimmune syndromes: an overview. Semin Arthritis Rheum 1999;28(6):392–7.

10. El-Hallak M, Giani T, Yeniay BS, et al. Chronic minocycline-induced autoimmunity in children. J Pediatr 2008;153:314–9.

11. Eshki M, Allanore L, Musette P, et al. Twelve-year analysis of severe cases of drug reaction with eosinophilia and systemic symptoms: a cause of unpredictable multiorgan failure. Arch Dermatol 2009;145:67–72.

12. Maubec E, Wolkenstein P, Loriot MA, et al. Minocycline-induced DRESS: evidence for accumulation of the culprit drug. Dermatology 2008;216: 200–4.

13. Shapiro LE, Knowles SR, Shear NH. Comparative safety of tetracycline, minocycline, and doxycycline. Arch Dermatol 1997;133(10):1224–30.

14. Berger RS. A double-blind, multiple-dose, placebo-controlled, cross-over study to compare the incidence of gastrointestinal complaints in healthy subjects given Doryx R and Vibramycin R. J Clin Pharmacol 1988;28:367–70.

15. Story MJ, McCloud PI, Boehm G. Doxycycline tolerance study. Incidence of nausea after doxycycline administration to healthy volunteers: a comparison of 2 formulations (Doryx vs Vibramycin). Eur J Clin Pharmacol 1991;40:419–21.

16. Jarvinen A, Nykanen S, Paasiniemi L, et al. Enteric coating reduces upper gastrointestinal adverse reactions to doxycycline. Clin Drug Invest 1995; 10(6):323–7.

17. Weinstein M, Laxer R, Debosz J, et al. Doxycycline-induced cutaneous inflammation with systemic symptoms in a patient with acne vulgaris. J Cutan Med Surg 2013;17(4):283–6.

18. Tabibian JH, Gutierrez MA. Doxycycline-induced pseudotumor cerebri. South Med J 2009;102(3): 310–1.

19. Friedman DI, Gordon LK, Egan RA, et al. Doxycycline and intracranial hypertension. Neurology 2004;62:2297–9.

20. Robles DT, Leonard JL, Compton N, et al. Severe drug hypersensitivity reaction in a young woman treated with doxycycline. Dermatology 2008;217: 23–6.

21. Mailhol C, Tremeau-Martinage C, Paul C, et al. Severe drug hypersensitivity reaction (DRESS syndrome) to doxycycline. Ann Dermatol Venereol 2010;137:40–3 [in French].

22. Meynadier J, Alirezai M. Systemic antibiotics for acne. Dermatology 1998;196:135–9.

23. Tan HH. Antibacterial therapy for acne. A guide to selection and use of systemic agents. Am J Clin Dermatol 2003;4(5):307–14.

24. Matsuura T, Shimizu Y, Fujimoto H, et al. Minocycline related lupus [letter]. Lancet 1992;340: 1553.

25. Sturkenboom MC, Meier CR, Jick H, et al. Minocycline and lupuslike syndrome in acne patients. Arch Intern Med 1999;159:493–7.

26. Schlienger RG, Bircher AJ, Meier CR. Minocycline-induced lupus: a systematic review. Dermatology 2000;200(3):223–31.

27. Seaman HE, Lawrenson RA, Williams TJ, et al. The risk of liver damage associated with minocycline: a comparative study. J Clin Pharmacol 2001;41(8): 852–60.

28. Christodoulou CS, Emmanuel P, Ray RA, et al. Respiratory distress due to minocycline-induced pulmonary lupus. Chest 1999;115(5):1471–3.

29. Edwards R. Doxycycline and photosensitivity [letter]. N Z Med J 1987;100:640.

30. Trueb RM, Burg G. Acute generalized exanthematous pustulosis due to doxycycline. Dermatology 1993;186:75–8.

31. Shaw JC. Antiandrogen and hormonal treatment of acne. Dermatol Clin 1996;14:803–11.

32. Goodfellow A, Alaghband-Zadeh J, Carter G, et al. Oral spironolactone improves acne vulgaris and reduces sebum excretion. Br J Dermatol 1984;111: 209–14.

33. Burke BM, Cunliffe WJ. Oral spironolactone therapy for female patients with acne, hirsutism or androgenic alopecia [letter]. Br J Dermatol 1985; 112:124–5.

34. Muhlemann MF, Carter GD, Cream JJ, et al. Oral spironolactone: an effective treatment for acne vulgaris in women. Br J Dermatol 1986;115:227–32.

35. Shaw JC. Spironolactone in dermatologic therapy. J Am Acad Dermatol 1991;24:236–43.

36. Hughes BR, Cunliffe WJ. Tolerance of spironolactone. Br J Dermatol 1988;118:687–91.

37. Shaw JC. Low-dose adjunctive spironolactone in the treatmet of acne in women: a retrospective analysis of 85 consecutively treated patients. J Am Acad Dermatol 2000;43:498–502.

38. Yemisci A, Gorgulu A, Piskin S. Effects and side-effects of spironolactone therapy in women with acne. J Eur Acad Dermatol Venereol 2005;19:163–6.

39. De Leo V, Morgante G. Different effectiveness of cyproterone acetate doses in treatment of acne. Clin Endocrinol 2003;58:246–7.

40. Plovanich M, Weng QY, Mostaghimi A. Low usefulness of potassium monitoring among healthy young women taking spironolactone for acne. JAMA Dermatol 2015;151(9):941–4.

41. Lubbos HG, Hasinski S, Rose LI, et al. Adverse effects of spironolactone therapy in women with acne. Arch Dermatol 1998;134(9):1162–3.

42. Cunliffe WJ, Simpson NB. Disorders of the sebaceous glands. In: Champion RH, Burton JL, Burns DA, et al, editors. Rook/Wilkinson/Ebling textbook of dermatology. 6th edition. Oxford (United Kingdom): Blackwell Science; 1998. p. 1927–84.

43. Brito MFM, Pessoa IS, Galindo JCS, et al. Evaluation of clinical adverse effects and laboratory alterations in patients with acne vulgaris treated with oral isotretinoin. An Bras Dermatol 2010;85(3): 331–6.

44. Orfanos CE, Zouboulis CC, Almond-Roesler B, et al. Current use and future potential role of retinoid drugs in dermatology. Drugs 1997;53:358–88.

45. Peck GL, DiGiovanna JJ. The retinoids. In: Freedberg IM, Eisen AZ, Wolff K, et al, editors. Dermatology in general medicine, vol. 2, 5th edition. New York: McGraw-Hill; 1999. p. 2810–20.

46. Sampaio SPA, Rivitti EA. Dermatologia. São Paulo (Brazil): Artes Médicas; 2001.

47. Azulay RD, Azulay DR. Dermatologia. Rio de Janeiro (Brazil): Guanabara Koogan; 2004.

48. Neudorfer M, Goldshtein I, Shamai-Lubovitz O, et al. Ocular adverse effects of systemic treatment with isotretinoin. Arch Dermatol 2012;148(7):803–8.

49. Fraunfelder FT, Fraunfelder FW, Edwards R. Ocular side effects possibly associated with isotretinoin usage. Am J Ophthalmol 2001;132(3):299–305.

50. Lerman S. Ocular side effects of accutane therapy. Lens Eye Toxic Res 1992;9:429–38.

51. Hanson N, Leachman S. Safety issues in isotretinoin therapy. Semin Cutan Med Surg 2001;20(3): 166–83.

52. Exner JH, Dahod S, Pochi PE. Pyogenic granuloma like acne lesions during isotretinoin therapy. Arch Dermatol 1983;119:808–11.

53. Schulpis KH, Georgala S, Papakonstantinou ED, et al. The effect of isotretinoin on biotinidase activity. Skin Pharmacol Appl Skin Physiol 1999; 12:28–33.

54. Ruiz-Maldonado R, Tamayo-Sanchez L, Orozco-Covarrubias ML. The use of retinoids in the pediatric patient. Dermatol Clin 1998;16:553–69.

55. Roche Laboratories Inc. Accutane (isotretinoin) capsules, in physicians' desk reference. 54th edition. Montvale (NJ): Medical Economics Company, Inc; 2000. p. 2610–2.

56. Rubenstein R, Roenigk HH Jr, Stegman SJ, et al. Atypical keloids after dermabrasion of patients taking isotretinoin. J Am Acad Dermatol 1986;15: 280–5.

57. Zachariae H. Delayed wound healing and keloid formation following argon laser treatment or dermabrasion during isotretinoin treatment. Br J Dermatol 1988;118:703–6.

58. Keller KL, Fenske NA. Uses of vitamins A, C, and E and related compounds in dermatology: a review. J Am Acad Dermatol 1998;39:611–25.

59. Ling TC, Parkin G, Islam J, et al. What is the cumulative effects or long-term, low-dose isotretinoin on the development of DISH? Br J Dermatol 2001;144: 630–702.

60. Milstone LM, McGuire J, Ablow RC. Premature epiphyseal closure in a child receiving oral 13-cis-retinoic acid. J Am Acad Dermatol 1982;7:663–6.

61. Heudes AM, Laroche L. Muscular damage during isotretinoin treatment. Ann Dermatol Venereol 1998;125:94–7.

62. Oikarinen A, Vuori J, Autio P, et al. Comparison of muscle-derived serum carbonic anhydrase III and myoglobin in dermatological patients: effects of isotretinoin treatment. Acta Derm Venereol 1992; 72:352–4.

63. Aurousseau MH, Levacher S, Beneton C, et al. Transient dysfibrinogenemia and thrombocytopenia associated with recurrent acute pancreatitis in the course of isotretinoin therapy. Rev Med Interne 1995;16:622–5.

64. Azon-Masoliver A, Grau C. Acute appendicitis and isotretinoin: a coincidence? J Eur Acad Dermatol Venereol 2000;14:233–4.

65. Amichai B, Grunwald MH, Odes SH, et al. Acute esophagitis caused by isotretinoin. Int J Dermatol 1996;35:528–9.

66. Prokop LD. Isotretinoin: possible component cause of inflammatory bowel disease. Am J Gastroenterol 1999;94:2568.

67. Godfrey KM, James MP. Treatment of severe acne with isotretinoin in patients with inflammatory bowel disease. Br J Dermatol 1990;123:653–5.

68. Adams J, Lammer EJ. Neurobehavioral tertology of isotretinoin. Reprod Toxicol 1998;7:175–7.

69. Maclean H, Wright M, Choi D, et al. Abnormal night vision with isotretinoin therapy for acne. Clin Exp Dermatol 1995;20:86.

70. Askmark H, Lundberg PO, Olsson S. Drug-related headache. Headache 1989;29:441–4.

71. Fisher DA. Exercise-induced bronchoconstriction related to isotretinoin therapy. J Am Acad Dermatol 1985;13:524.

72. Kapur N, Hughes JR, Rustin MH. Exacerbation of asthma by isotretinoin. Br J Dermatol 2000;142:388–9.

73. RxList.com [homepage]. Available at: http://www.rxlist.com/cgi/generic/isotret_ad.htm. Accessed August 12, 2014.

74. Pavese P, Kuentz F, Belleville C, et al. Renal impairment induced by isotretinoin. Nephrol Dial Transplant 1997;12:1299.

75. Edwards S, Sonnex C. Urethritis associated with isotretinoin therapy. Acta Derm Venereol 1997;77:330.

76. Lamberg L. Acne drug depression warnings highlight need for expert care. JAMA 1998;279:1057.

77. Wysowski DK, Pitts M, Beitz J. Depression and suicide in patients treated with isotretinoin. N Engl J Med 2001;344:460.

78. Magin P, Pond D, Smith W. Isotretinoin, depression and suicide: a review of evidence. Br J Gen Pract 2005;55:134–8.

79. Jick SS, Kremers HM, Vasilakis-Scaramozza C. Isotretinoin use and risk of depression, psychotic symptoms, suicide, and attempted suicide. Arch Dermatol 2001;137:1102–3.

80. Chu A, Cunliffe WJ. The inter-relationship between isotretinoin/acne and depression. J Eur Acad Dermatol Venereol 1999;12:263.

81. McLane J. Analysis of common side effects of isotretinoin. J Am Acad Dermatol 2001;45:S188–94.

82. Kamm JJ. Toxicology, carcinogenicity, and teratogenicity of some orally administered retinoids. J Am Acad Dermatol 1982;6:652–9.

83. Roenigk HH Jr. Liver toxicity of retinoid therapy. J Am Acad Dermatol 1988;19:199–208.

84. Nguyen EH, Wolverton SE. Systemic retinoids. In: Wolverton SE, editor. Comprehensive dermatologic drug therapy. Philadelphia: Saunders; 2001. p. 269–310.

85. Vahlquist C, Michaelsson G, Vahlquist A, et al. A sequential comparison of etretinate (Tigason) and isotretinoin (Roaccutane) with special regard to their effects on serum lipoproteins. Br J Dermatol 1985;112:69–76.

86. American academy of pediatrics committee on drugs: retinoid therapy for severe dermatological disorders. Pediatrics 1992;90:119–20.

87. Flynn WJ, Freeman PG, Wickboldt LG. Pancreatitis associated with isotretinoin-induced hypertriglyceridemia. Ann Intern Med 1987;107:63.

88. Michaelsson G, Vahlquist A, Mobacken H, et al. Changes in laboratory variables induced by isotretinoin treatment of acne. Acta Derm Venereol 1986;66:144–8.

89. Williams RE, Doherty VR, Perkins W, et al. Staphylococcus aureus and intranasal mupicorin in patients receiving isotretinoin for acne. Br J Dermatol 1992;126:362–4.

90. Patton TJ, Zirwas MJ, Wolverton SE. Systemic retinoids. In: Wolverton SE, editor. Comprehensive dermatologic drug therapy. 2nd edition. Philadelphia: Saunders; 2007. p. 276–95.

91. Batra RS. Acne. In: Kenneth AA, Hsu JTS, editors. Manual of dermatologic therapeutics. 7th edition. Philadelphia: Lippincott Williams & Wilkins; 2007. p. 3–17.

92. Kaymak Y, Iler N. The effectiveness of intermittent isotretinoin treatment in mild or moderate acne. J Eur Acad Dermatol Venereol 2006;20:1256–60.

93. Akman A, Durusoy C, Senturk M, et al. Treatment of acne with intermittent and conventional isotretinoin: a randomized, controlled multicenter study. Arch Dermatol Res 2007;299:467–73.

94. Amchai B, Shemer A, Grunwald MH. Low-dose isotretinoin in the treatment of acne vulgaris. J Am Acad Dermatol 2006;54:644–6.

95. Sardana K, Garg VK, Sehgal VN, et al. Efficacy of fixed low-dose isotretinoin (20 mg, alternate days) with topical clindamycin gel in moderately severe acne vulgaris. J Eur Acad Dermatol Venereol 2009;23:556–60.

96. Kumar CA, Kumar CVK. Toxicity of low-dose intermittent isotretinoin in recalcitrant acne. Med J Armed Forces India 2010;66:208–12.

97. Altman RS, Altman LJ, Altman JS. A proposed set of new guidelines for routine blood tests during isotretinoin therapy for acne vulgaris. Dermatology 2002;204:232–5.

98. Tallab T, Joharji H, Jazei M, et al. Isotretinoin therapy: any need for laboratory assessment? West Afr J Med 2004;23:273–5.

99. Ellis CN, Krach KJ. Uses and complications of isotretinoin therapy. J Am Acad Dermatol 2001;45:S150–7.

100. Alcalay J, Landau M, Zucker A. Analysis of laboratory data in acne patients treated with isotretinoin: is there really a need to perform routine laboratory tests? J Dermatolog Treat 2001;12:9–12.

101. Leachman SA, Insogna KL, Katz L, et al. Bone densities in patients receiving isotretinoin for cystic acne. Arch Dermatol 1999;135:961–5.

Pediatric Acne
Clinical Patterns and Pearls

Lidia Maroñas-Jiménez, MD[a], Andrew C. Krakowski, MD[b,c],*

KEYWORDS

- Neonatal • Infantile • Midchildhood • Preadolescent • Acne • Treatment • Adherence • Evaluation

KEY POINTS

- Neonatal acne, which may be clinically distinct from neonatal cephalic pustulosis, can present with true comedones.
- Infantile acne has the potential to cause scarring and may be a predictor of more severe adolescent acne.
- Midchildhood acne (ages 1–7 years) may herald the presence of a hyperandrogenic state (eg, underlying tumor, adrenal enzyme deficiency) and warrants prompt evaluation.
- Preadolescent acne presents at around 7 to 12 years of age; it is usually considered normal and may be the first sign of pubertal maturation.

INTRODUCTION

Rare is the patient who achieves adulthood without having had some degree of acne.[1,2] Although the prevalence of acne may reach 95% in the adolescent population, acne should not be considered solely a teenage problem.[3,4] In a poster presentation at the American Academy of Dermatology Annual Meeting (Boston, MA, August 2012), Sandoval and colleagues reported, as part of the National Ambulatory Medical Care Data Survey, some 55 million pediatric acne visits in a 6-year period. The data showed that neonatal/infantile acne compromised approximately 3% of visits overall; midchildhood acne accounted for 0.9% of cases; and preadolescent acne constituted 4.8% of total acne visits. In contrast with neonatal acne, for which pediatricians treated approximately 75% of cases, pediatricians and dermatologists treated preadolescent acne cases almost equally (38% and 34% of cases, respectively).

Managing patients with pediatric acne can be a challenge in daily clinical practice. The wide spectrum of differential diagnoses, the possibility of underlying systemic disorders, and the potential for side effects from medications demand vigilance and should incite humility from even the most seasoned acneologist. However, acne management in this population comes with great reward for patients and providers alike. This article provides a practical approach to acne, reviewing the current perspectives on underlying causes, evaluation, and treatment from birth to preadolescence (**Fig. 1**).

PEDIATRIC PHYSIOLOGY

The stereotypical timing of pediatric acne onset reflects physiologic changes that normally occur as people develop from fetus to teenager. Starting in utero and continuing until about the first 6 to 12 months of life, both boys and girls produce high levels of dehydroepiandrosterone (DHEA) and its sulfated form (DHEAS), the result of a prominent zona reticularis in the fetal adrenal glands, which leads to stimulation of sebaceous

[a] Department of Dermatology, Hospital Universitario 12 de Octubre, Medical School, Universidad Complutense, Institute i+12, Avenida de Córdoba s/n, Madrid 28041, Spain; [b] Division of Pediatric and Adolescent Dermatology, Rady Children's Hospital, 8010 Frost Street, Suite 602, San Diego, CA 92123, USA; [c] DermOne, LLC, Four Tower Bridge, 200 Barr Harbor Drive, Suite 200, West Conshohocken, PA 19428, USA
* Corresponding author. Division of Pediatric and Adolescent Dermatology, Rady Children's Hospital, San Diego, CA.
E-mail address: ackrakowski@gmail.com

Dermatol Clin 34 (2016) 195–202
http://dx.doi.org/10.1016/j.det.2015.11.006
0733-8635/16/$ – see front matter © 2016 Elsevier Inc. All rights reserved.

derm.theclinics.com

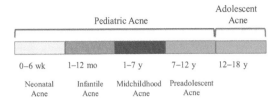

Fig. 1. Approximate age of onset of various pediatric acne types.

glands.[5] In addition, boys during this time show increasing levels of luteinizing hormone (LH) and secrete high levels of testicular testosterone, helping to explain why acne occurs more frequently in boys than in girls during the first year of life.[6–12] At around 1 year of age, hormonal activity decreases with progressive involution of the fetal adrenal glands, highlighting that new-onset or persistent acne in this age group warrants evaluation for a more serious underlying medical disorder. With normal onset of adrenarche at around 7 years of age, DHEAS levels increase once again. This change correlates with the emergence of preadolescent acne, which may be the first sign of pubertal maturation.[13,14]

NEONATAL ACNE

Neonatal acne may be present at birth or appear shortly thereafter, usually during the first 4 to 6 weeks of life (Table 1).[15] Most commonly seen in boys, neonatal acne has been reported to affect up to 20% of newborns, although it is not certain that all these eruptions are true acne.[5,8,9] Clinical presentation within this age group is likely associated with several causal factors: increased sebum production, hormonal stimulation of sebaceous glands by both maternal (primarily through the placenta rather than via lactation) and neonatal androgens, and colonization of sebaceous glands by lipophilic species of the genus Malassezia.[5,6]

The presence of small closed comedones typically limited to the face (forehead, nose, and cheeks) confirms the diagnosis of true neonatal acne. These acneiform lesions may progress to more extensive inflammatory forms with erythematous papules, pustules, and scarring cysts over the neck and upper trunk (Fig. 2).[5,16,17]

A topical retinoid with or without benzoyl peroxide is typically all that is needed to help treat true neonatal acne. Referral to a pediatric dermatologist is warranted if acneiform lesions persist, especially in the clinical setting of scarring. In those rare cases when the diagnosis is unclear, a thorough family history helps to rule out an underlying acneiform drug reaction, and laboratory investigations may occasionally be required to exclude infectious causes.[6,16–18] When an underlying cause of true virilization, such as congenital adrenal hyperplasia or virilizing tumor, is suspected a careful physical examination that includes developmental and growth parameters, blood pressure, and investigation for additional signs of hyperandrogenism, like precocious sexual maturation, should be performed.[6,10,14,17–19] Complementary work-up assessing adrenal function and androgen excess with DHEAS and free

Table 1 Neonatal acne	
Differential Diagnosis	Neonatal cephalic pustulosis; infectious agents; transient neonatal pustular melanosis; nevus comedonicus; erythema toxicum neonatorum; sebaceous gland hyperplasia; milia; miliaria; maternal medications (eg, lithium, phenytoin, corticosteroids); congenital adrenal hyperplasia; virilizing tumor; other underlying endocrinopathy
Age at Onset	In utero to ~6 wk
Morphology	Comedones Inflammatory papules Pustules Nodules/cysts Scarring
Distribution	Forehead Cheeks Nose Less commonly: neck, chest, back
Clinical Pearls	• Tends to resolve spontaneously • Topical retinoids may be helpful • Consider referral to a pediatric dermatologist if lesions persist or scarring becomes a concern

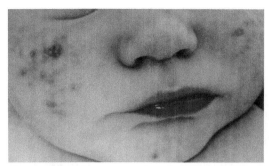

Fig. 2. A 4-week-old boy with neonatal acne on bilateral cheeks and chin; note the presence of true closed comedones along with inflammatory papules and pustules.

testosterone, usually directed by or in conjunction with pediatric endocrinology, is recommended in these rare cases.[14,17,19]

Differentiating true neonatal acne from the entity called neonatal cephalic pustulosis (NCP) remains controversial, because the two terms have historically and confusingly been used interchangeably.[16,19] NCP generally appears within the first several weeks of life as a mild inflammatory papulopustular eruption, primarily localizing to the forehead, eyelids, cheeks, and chin; less commonly, NCP may also involve the scalp, neck, chest, and upper back.[17,19] NCP has been reported to be a transient disorder that occurs in up to 25% of newborns and often resolves spontaneously, typically without scarring, in days to weeks.[18–20] The absence of true comedones, either closed or open, in NCP is a useful distinctive clinical feature.[19]

Malassezia species (*Malassezia furfur*, *Malassezia globosa*, and *Malassezia sympodialis*), a normal flora of infant skin, have long been suspected of playing a causative role in the development of NCP. Given the presence of this yeast in lesional skin smears of affected infants, some studies suggest an association between cutaneous colonization with *Malassezia* and the pustular condition in newborns.[21,22] However, not all patients with NCP have positive microbiological findings for *Malassezia*.[23] In addition, not all culture-positive neonates develop NCP-like skin lesions.[24] Ayhan and colleagues[25] found no significant differences in skin colonization with *Malassezia* between patients with NCP and healthy neonates. One plausible explanation for these findings is that NCP may be a hypersensitivity response to the presence of the yeast in predisposed individuals rather than a pathologic disease caused by an increase in the number of microorganisms.[22,23,25] Alternatively, other pustular eruptions of the neonate may present similarly to *Malassezia*-associated NCP, which may confound the reported results.

Because of its typical self-limited course, aggressive treatment of NCP is often not required.[26] Application of topical ketoconazole cream has been reported to expedite clearance of lesions and reduce fungal colonization; however, more rigorous investigations are necessary before formal, evidence-based recommendations can be made.[6,14,17,18,21]

INFANTILE ACNE

Infantile acne typically begins between 6 weeks to 1 year of life (**Table 2**).[19,27] Lesions consist of closed and open comedones, inflammatory papules, and pustules, primarily localizing to the face and, less commonly, to the chest and back. Severe cysts leading to scarring may be present (**Fig. 3**).[12,17,28] Exceptional cases of acne

Table 2 Infantile acne	
Differential Diagnosis	Infectious agents (eg, molluscum contagiosum); periorificial dermatitis; keratosis pilaris; exogenous causes (eg, acne pomade, chloracne, steroid acne)
Age at Onset	~4–6 wk to 1 y
Morphology	Comedones Inflammatory papules (may resemble abscesses) Pustules Nodules/cysts Scarring
Distribution	Face (cheeks prominently affected) Chest Back
Clinical Pearls	• Routine cultures of lesions are sterile • Signs such as testicular enlargement or pubic hair signal possible precocious puberty • Scarring may require isotretinoin • May predict more severe adolescent acne

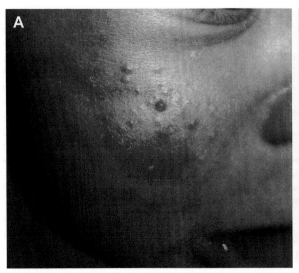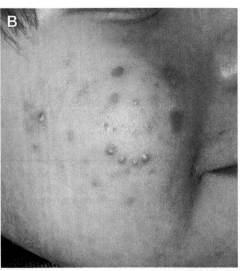

Fig. 3. (A) A 4-month-old boy with infantile acne at risk for scarring. After failing topical therapies, oral erythromycin was initiated; the family deferred isotretinoin. (B) The patient 3 months later with notable improvement but evidence of mild scarring.

conglobata with large sinus tracts and keloid scars have also been reported among this age group.[5,7] More than 80% of patients experience only a mild to moderate course that resolves spontaneously by 1 or 2 years of age; however, infantile acne may have an unpredictable course with active lesions lasting for several years, even up to puberty, and may be a predictor of more severe adolescent acne.[6–8,12,16–18,27]

The exact cause of infantile acne has yet to be elucidated. The condition is more common in boys, supporting the role of increased sensitivity of sebaceous glands to circulating androgens (caused by midpubertal testicular levels of androgens as well as the higher levels of adrenal androgens seen in both sexes).[5,7,12,17] Some cases with a positive family history of severe acne suggest the importance of a predisposing genetic background.[7,19]

Although most patients with infantile acne do not require extensive evaluation, several reports have described an association with underlying hormonal abnormalities, including increased levels of testosterone, LH, and follicle-stimulating hormone (FSH), and, rarely, adrenocortical malignancies.[29,30] The general diagnostic approach should systematically include clinical evaluation of possible physical manifestations secondary to corticosteroid-secreting or androgen-secreting disorders.[7,14,17,18] Children whose clinical examination is suggestive of hyperandrogenism (eg, pubic hair, testicular enlargement), as well as those in whom acne is severe or recalcitrant, may require further evaluation

with bone age assessment; serologic determination of at least LH, FSH, free testosterone, and DHEAS levels; and referral to a pediatric endocrinologist.[14] Rapid onset of acne may warrant additional investigations to exclude the possibility of a virilizing tumor.[5] Close follow-up of patients with infantile acne through childhood is recommended for early detection of persistent disease, which is considered to be an indicator of possible underlying endocrinopathy.[18]

Infantile acne is essentially treated like acne at any age. The absence of randomized controlled trials and the lack of US Food and Drug Administration–approved acne medications for children less than 9 years of age mean that the therapeutic approach to these patients is empirically based on observations in adults and adolescents.[14,27,31] Benzoyl peroxide and topical retinoids may be used as monotherapy or in combination.[14,18] Burning, stinging, scaling, and dryness are the most common side effects and may be mitigated by decreasing the frequency of use to alternate days, initiating treatment at a lower potency, applying smaller amounts of medication, and using noncomedogenic moisturizers regularly.[14,27] Inflammatory lesions may be treated with topical antibiotics (eg, clindamycin, erythromycin, or a combination product). In severe inflammatory cases or when scarring is evident or is a developing concern, treatment with systemic antibiotics may be warranted. Oral erythromycin is an excellent first choice unless patients have known *Propionibacterium acnes* resistance, in which case oral sulfamethoxazole-trimethoprim may be a better option. Tetracyclines should be avoided because of the risk of permanent tooth staining. Isolated deep nodules and cysts can be treated with intralesional injections of triamcinolone at a low concentration (2.5 mg/mL) to decrease the risk of systemic absorption and cutaneous atrophy at the sites of injection.[6,17,19]

Children with recalcitrant, scarring acne may require oral isotretinoin to prevent long-term physical and psychological impact of the disease.[14] Off-label use of isotretinoin in infants and younger children with severe acne has been well documented in the literature.[24,28,31,32] Most published infantile cases have reported safe treatments with doses ranging from 0.2 to 2 mg/kg/d for 4 to 14 months.[6,27] Isotretinoin may be given in 2 daily doses, hidden within a candy bar after freezing and cutting a capsule into proper doses, or within a spoonful of warm milk after opening the capsule in dim light.[17] Close clinical and laboratory monitoring in these patients is recommended, similar to treatment in the adolescent and adult populations.

MIDCHILDHOOD ACNE

Midchildhood acne, the rarest form of acne, is a cause for alarm (Table 3). It typically has its onset between 1 and 7 years of age and is clinically characterized by the presence of mixed comedonal and inflammatory lesions over the face.[14] Because adrenal secretion virtually ceases after the first year of life and remains quiescent until around 6 to 8 years of age, the appearance of true acne in this age group raises concern for underlying causes of hyperandrogenemia (eg, true precocious puberty, Cushing syndrome, late-onset congenital adrenal hyperplasia, adrenal or gonadal androgen-secreting tumors).[5–7,14,17,19]

Full physical examination, including evaluation of the growth chart to make sure that height is not accelerating across percentiles (androgen excess) or slowing down (Cushing syndrome) is necessary. Bone age may be assessed by plain radiograph of the left hand and wrist. Serologic work-up may include free testosterone, DHEAS, LH, FSH, prolactin, and 17α-hydroxyprogesterone. If adrenal tumors or Cushing syndrome are suspected, then an adrenocorticotropic hormone (ACTH) stimulation test, serum ACTH levels, and a 24-hour urinary cortisol test may be helpful. Because of the severe implications of acne in this age group, referral to a pediatric endocrinologist is recommended.[5,14] Treatment in this age group focuses on addressing the underlying cause. If patients require additional management of their acne, then the approach should parallel that of infantile acne.

PREADOLESCENT ACNE

Preadolescent is defined by the appearance of acne vulgaris in children 7 to 12 years of age (Table 4).[14] Clinically, the earliest lesions of preadolescent acne are typically comedones affecting the central forehead. Lesions gradually evolve to inflammatory papules and pustules, involving the center of the face and, possibly, the conchae of the ears. Lesions may spread to the jawline, lateral cheeks, chest, back, and neck.

Although acne in this age group is usually normal, it may be a sign of an underlying problem such as late-onset congenital adrenal hyperplasia or polycystic ovary syndrome. Management algorithms in this age group are well documented and parallel adolescent and adult strategies. However, treatment success may be thwarted by the

Table 3 Midchildhood acne	
Differential Diagnosis	Underlying hyperandrogenic state; flat warts; demodicosis; molluscum contagiosum; periorificial dermatitis; pityrosporum folliculitis; pseudoacne of the nasal crease; idiopathic facial aseptic granuloma; keratosis pilaris
Age at Onset	1–7 y
Morphology	Comedones Inflammatory papules Pustules
Distribution	Face Chest Back
Clinical Pearls	• Acne is rare in this age group • Growth charts are helpful assessment tools • May herald presence of hyperandrogenic state • Prompt evaluation and/or referral to pediatric endocrinologist is warranted

Table 4 Preadolescent acne	
Differential Diagnosis	Flat warts; demodicosis; molluscum contagiosum; periorificial dermatitis; pityrosporum folliculitis; pseudoacne of the nasal crease; idiopathic facial aseptic granuloma; keratosis pilaris
Age at Onset	~7–12 y
Morphology	Comedones Inflammatory papules Pustules Nodules/cysts
Distribution	Face (especially forehead) Conchae of ears may be involved Chest Back
Clinical Pearls	• Incidence is increasing with decreasing age of puberty • Consider possibility of underlying condition such as polycystic ovary syndrome or late-onset congenital adrenal hyperplasia • Treatment is similar to adolescent and adult algorithms but "less may be more" (i.e., a less complicated regimen with minimal side effects) in this preteen population

combination of unmotivated preteen patients and regimens that are too complicated. Consequently, it may be helpful to involve the parents directly in the acne plan and to keep recommendations for treatment as simple as possible, with tolerability and ease of application in mind.

More related to pubertal development than to age, preadolescent acne reflects the physiologic awakening of adrenal glands, which usually occurs at 6 to 7 years in girls and 7 to 8 years in boys.[33,34] Accordingly, levels of DHEA and DHEAS start increasing, and sebaceous gland secretion reactivates.[35] Several studies have shown that girls with severe comedonal acne have higher levels of DHEAS compared with girls with no acne or mild comedonal acne, with the biggest difference between these two groups occurring 2 years before menarche.[36] In addition, it has been reported that increases in sebum production and P acnes colonization occur in parallel in children with acne from the age of 8 years; colonization rates in the nares correlated prospectively with age, whereas skin colonization correlated with pubertal status and presence of acne.[37] Together these studies support the notion that high levels of DHEAS at an earlier stage of development may be associated with earlier onset of sebum production and that acne-prone children may secrete sebum earlier than children without acne, allowing earlier colonization by P acnes.

The epidemiologic profile of preadolescent acne continues to evolve. In 1994, Lucky and colleagues[38] reported acne lesions in almost 80% of 365 girls aged 9 to 10 years, and more recent demographic research supports the presence of the condition in 7-year-old to 11-year-old patients in the United States.[39] Clearly, 12+ years of age is no longer the lower end of normal acne onset.[40] The current trend toward a decreasing age of puberty onset in the Western world may help explain the increasing incidence of preadolescent acne.[27,40]

SUMMARY

Diagnosis and management of pediatric acne in any age group begins with a careful history and physical examination and a general awareness of normal physiology. Medical intervention should begin with the least aggressive topical treatment regimen that targets as many age-appropriate pathogenic factors as possible. Once treatment has been implemented, clinicians must be willing to ramp up to systemic therapies whenever necessary to prevent acne-related scarring, just as they would for their adolescent and adult patients. Treatment-specific side effects should be anticipated and discussed with patients and their families, using education as its own distinct acne intervention. In certain age groups, especially midchildhood patients, clinicians must recognize that acne may herald an underlying disorder. Prompt consultation with another specialist, such as a pediatric endocrinologist or pediatric dermatologist, is warranted in these rare but serious cases.

REFERENCES

1. Collier CN, Harper JC, Cafardi JA, et al. The prevalence of acne in adults 20 years and older. J Am Acad Dermatol 2008;58(1):56–9.

2. Knutsen-Larson S, Dawson AL, Dunnick CA, et al. Acne vulgaris: pathogenesis, treatment, and needs assessment. Dermatol Clin 2012;30(1):99–106.

3. Dreno B, Poli F. Epidemiology of acne. Dermatology 2003;206(1):7–10.

4. Cordain L, Lindeberg S, Hurtado M, et al. Acne vulgaris: a disease of Western civilization. Arch Dermatol 2002;138(12):1584–90.

5. Tom WL, Friedlander SF. Acne through the ages: case-based observations through childhood and adolescence. Clin Pediatr 2008;47(7):639–51.

6. Antoniou C, Dessinioti C, Stratigos AJ, et al. Clinical and therapeutic approach to childhood acne: an update. Pediatr Dermatol 2009;26(4):373–80.

7. Herane MI, Ando I. Acne in infancy and acne genetics. Dermatology 2003;206(1):24–8.

8. Jansen T, Burgdorf WH, Plewig G. Pathogenesis and treatment of acne in childhood. Pediatr Dermatol 1997;14(1):17–21.

9. Yonkosky DM, Pochi PE. Acne vulgaris in childhood: pathogenesis and management. Dermatol Clin 1986;4(1):127–36.

10. Katsambas AD, Katoulis AC, Stavropoulos P. Acne neonatorum: a study of 22 cases. Int J Dermatol 1999;38(2):128–30.

11. Shaw JC. Acne: effect of hormones on pathogenesis and management. Am J Clin Dermatol 2002;3(8):571–8.

12. Cunliffe WJ, Baron SE, Coulson IH. A clinical and therapeutic study of 29 patients with infantile acne. Br J Dermatol 2001;145(3):463–6.

13. Fried RG, Webster GF, Eichenfield LF, et al. Medical and psychosocial impact of acne. Semin Cutan Med Surg 2010;29(2 Suppl 1):9–12.

14. Eichenfield LF, Krakowski AC, Piggott C, et al. Evidence-based recommendations for the diagnosis and treatment of pediatric acne. Pediatrics 2013;131(Suppl 3):S163–86.

15. Nanda S, Reddy BS, Ramji S, et al. Analytical study of pustular eruptions in neonates. Pediatr Dermatol 2002;19(3):210–5.

16. Serna-Tamayo C, Janniger CK, Micali G, et al. Neonatal and infantile acne vulgaris: an update. Cutis 2014;94(1):13–6.

17. Krakowski AC, Eichenfield LF. Pediatric acne: clinical presentations, evaluation, and management. J Drugs Dermatol 2007;6(6):589–93.

18. Friedlander SF, Baldwin HE, Mancini AJ, et al. The acne continuum: an age-based approach to therapy. Semin Cutan Med Surg 2011;30(3 Suppl):S6–11.

19. Cantatore-Francis JL, Glick SA. Childhood acne: evaluation and management. Dermatol Ther 2006;19(4):202–9.

20. Bardazzi F, Patrizi A. Transient cephalic neonatal pustulosis. Arch Dermatol 1997;133(4):528–30.

21. Rapelanoro R, Mortureux P, Couprie B, et al. Neonatal Malassezia furfur pustulosis. Arch Dermatol 1996;132(2):190–3.

22. Niamba P, Weill FX, Sarlangue J, et al. Is common neonatal cephalic pustulosis (neonatal acne) triggered by Malassezia sympodialis? Arch Dermatol 1998;134(8):995–8.

23. Bernier V, Weill FX, Hirigoyen V, et al. Skin colonization by Malassezia species in neonates: a prospective study and relationship with neonatal cephalic pustulosis. Arch Dermatol 2002;138(2):215–8.

24. Bergman JN, Eichenfield LF. Neonatal acne and cephalic pustulosis: is Malassezia the whole story? Arch Dermatol 2002;138(2):255–7.

25. Ayhan M, Sancak B, Karaduman A, et al. Colonization of neonate skin by Malassezia species: relationship with neonatal cephalic pustulosis. J Am Acad Dermatol 2007;57(6):1012–8.

26. Kaminer MS, Gilchrest BA. The many faces of acne. J Am Acad Dermatol 1995;32(5 Pt 3):S6–14.

27. Admani S, Barrio VR. Evaluation and treatment of acne from infancy to preadolescence. Dermatol Ther 2013;26(6):462–6.

28. Torrelo A, Pastor MA, Zambrano A. Severe acne infantum successfully treated with isotretinoin. Pediatr Dermatol 2005;22(4):357–9.

29. Duke EM. Infantile acne associated with transient increases in plasma concentrations of luteinising hormone, follicle-stimulating hormone, and testosterone. Br Med J (Clinical Res Ed) 1981;282(6272):1275–6.

30. Mann MW, Ellis SS, Mallory SB. Infantile acne as the initial sign of an adrenocortical tumor. J Am Acad Dermatol 2007;56(2 Suppl):S15–8.

31. Miller IM, Echeverria B, Torrelo A, et al. Infantile acne treated with oral isotretinoin. Pediatr Dermatol 2013;30(5):513–8.

32. Sarazin F, Dompmartin A, Nivot S, et al. Treatment of an infantile acne with oral isotretinoin. Eur J Dermatol 2004;14(1):71–2.

33. Ibáñez L, Dimartino-Nardi J, Potau N, et al. Premature adrenarche–normal variant or forerunner of adult disease? Endocr Rev 2000;21(6):671–96.

34. Kaplowitz PB, Oberfield SE. Reexamination of the age limit for defining when puberty is precocious in girls in the United States: implications for evaluation and treatment. Drug and Therapeutics and Executive Committees of the Lawson Wilkins Pediatric Endocrine Society. Pediatrics 1999;104(4 Pt 1):936–41.

35. Stewart ME, Downing DT, Cook JS, et al. Sebaceous gland activity and serum dehydroepiandrosterone sulfate levels in boys and girls. Arch Dermatol 1992;128(10):1345–8.

36. Lucky AW, Biro FM, Simbartl LA, et al. Predictors of severity of acne vulgaris in young adolescent girls:

results of a five-year longitudinal study. J Pediatr 1997;130(1):30–9.

37. Mourelatos K, Eady EA, Cunliffe WJ, et al. Temporal changes in sebum excretion and propionibacterial colonization in preadolescent children with and without acne. Br J Dermatol 2007; 156(1):22–31.

38. Lucky AW, Biro FM, Huster GA, et al. Acne vulgaris in premenarchal girls. An early sign of puberty associated with rising levels of dehydroepiandrosterone. Arch Dermatol 1994;130(3):308–14.

39. Mancini AJ, Baldwin HE, Eichenfield LF, et al. Acne life cycle: the spectrum of pediatric disease. Semin Cutan Med Surg 2011;30(3 Suppl): S2–5.

40. Friedlander SF, Eichenfield LF, Fowler JF Jr, et al. Acne epidemiology and pathophysiology. Semin Cutan Med Surg 2010;29(2 Suppl 1):2–4.

Evaluation and Management of Refractory Acne Vulgaris in Adolescent and Adult Men

Morgan McCarty, DO

KEYWORDS

- Acne • Sebum production • Transepidermal water loss • Male

KEY POINTS

- A male's normal skin physiologic state is different than a female's and may have implications when choosing treatment when the skin is altered in a disease state.
- Transepidermal water loss, pH, and sebum production are different between the sexes.
- Acne vulgaris alters the normal skin physiology, including impairment of the stratum corneum and transepidermal water loss.
- There are several underlying conditions presenting in male acne patients at several ages that may require a more in-depth evaluation.

Men are from Mars and women are from Venus,[1] but is this true when treating male patients with acne? Several skin physiologic variances exist between the sexes and may lead physicians to approach their male acne patients differently. Several aspects, including transepidermal water loss (TEWL), pH, and sebum production, have all been demonstrated to be different between the sexes. Adolescent and adult men are also more likely to be affected by seborrheic dermatitis, which shares a similar inflammatory cascade to acne pathogenesis and which may have therapeutic implications for acne. Adolescent and adult men may also consume supplements that increase their insulin growth factor-1 and predispose them to developing more acne. There are also several underlying conditions presenting with acne in adolescent and adult men in several age groups that may require further investigation. As more is learned about skin physiology and the pathogenesis of acne, these few baseline skin physiologic differences may in fact change the approach to male patients with acne in the future.

TEWL has recently become an important concept in dermatology and when approaching patients with acne.[2,3] According to Luebberding and colleagues,[1] in examination of 300 healthy men and women, TEWL was found to be significantly lower in the male cohort than the water loss of women in the same age category until age 50. The implications of this finding are important in the treatment of acne in adolescent male patients. Yamamoto and colleagues[2] demonstrated that patients with acne have impairment of the stratum corneum and TEWL. This impairment of the stratum corneum correlates with the burden of disease. If adolescent male patients begin with a baseline TEWL lower than adolescent female patients, and then develop moderate to severe acne that affects the normal baseline function of their stratum corneum, adolescent male patients in theory would deviate farther from their normal physiologic state and perhaps be more

Department of Dermatology, Baylor Scott & White, 409 West Adams, Temple, TX 76501, USA
E-mail address: morganmccarty@gmail.com

Dermatol Clin 34 (2016) 203–206
http://dx.doi.org/10.1016/j.det.2015.11.007
0733-8635/16/$ – see front matter © 2016 Elsevier Inc. All rights reserved.

prone to adverse side effects of acne therapies that augment barrier function more than female patients. Harper[4] demonstrated gender and age differences between male and female patients and found improved treatment success with clindamycin phosphate 1.2%/benzoyl peroxide 2.5% gel in young adolescent women and older adult men. The Harper study supports the differences outlined in the research of Luebberding and colleagues[1] of gender variance based on age of male and female patients, demonstrating TEWL becomes more similar with age. Nearly all of the medications used in the dermatology armamentarium augment barrier function, including benzoyl peroxide, topical retinoids, and isotretinoin.[3] However, if TEWL and stratum corneum function are maintained at near normal levels by the practitioner when treating male acne patients, medications that target key gender differences may improve outcomes in acne treatment. Preservation of TEWL and stratum corneum health is a target area for new therapeutic formulations in the future of acne treatment.

The pH of physiologically normal skin is 5.4. However, male patients have significantly lower pH values, less than 5.0, than female patients, which are higher than 5.0, regardless of age.[1] Free fatty acids are elevated in male skin because of higher production of sebum, causing the pH to be different from female patients. Although the implications of pH in acne pathogenesis have not yet been elucidated, as more is learned, the pH difference may have implications when developing appropriate acne treatment formulations for proper delivery of topical medications between the sexes.[5,6]

Sebum production is elevated in male patients in comparison with female patients.[3] Even though elevated sebum production alone does not induce acne, alterations in sebum composition have been demonstrated to cause follicular hypercornification via stimulation of the innate immune system directly and indirectly. Sebum also promotes an anaerobic environment for *Propionibacterium acnes* to thrive. *P acnes* is able to drive inflammatory cytokines through toll-like receptors 2 and 4 (TLR); this is followed by elevated production of interleukin (IL)-1β, which induces IL-6, IL-8, and IL-12. Eventual stimulation of activator protein-1 causes activation of matrix metalloproteinases (MMPs) and theoretic increase for scar formation.[7–12] Adolescent and adult men, in theory, are at increased risk of developing acne scarring based on elevated sebum production and upregulation of the inflammatory cascade compared with female acne patients (**Fig. 1**). Therefore, topical and oral retinoids may be even more beneficial in male patients because of their direct effect on the sebaceous gland activity, leading to a greater degree of reduction in sebum and inhibition of inflammation and eventual MMPs that cause scar formation.[12]

Seborrheic dermatitis is a chronic dermatitis that affects 5% of the population, with young men comprising a large proportion.[13] The male population overrepresentation is thought to be from excessive sebum compared with other affected cohorts. In the past, seborrheic dermatitis was

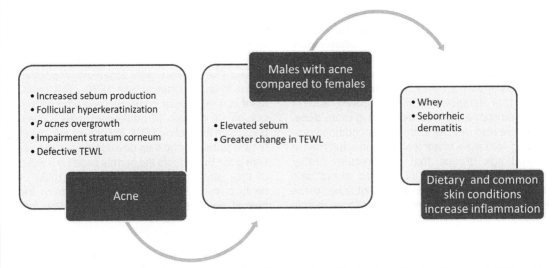

Fig. 1. The pathogenesis of acne and several unique features that affect male patients with acne. Additional influences that may affect male patients include dietary supplements and higher prevalence of seborrheic dermatitis.

thought to be solely from overgrowth of *Malassezia* species that flourish in more oil-prone areas. Recent data have discovered dandruff sufferers actually have a mixed bacterial and fungal imbalance that predisposes them to this chronic issue. One of the implicated bacterial species is *P acnes*.[14] Examination of the purposed inflammatory cascade of seborrheic dermatitis activates the innate immune stimulation by *Malassezia restricta* through the nodlike receptor 3 (NLRP3) on sebocytes that induce IL-1β.[15] The nodlike receptors are a class of pattern-recognition receptors similar in function to TLR. *P acnes* has also been demonstrated to activate this cascade through NLRP3. *P acnes*–induced inflammation is reduced in NLRP3-deficient mice.[16] Adolescent and adult men are more likely to suffer from seborrheic dermatitis, and this NLRP3 inflammatory cascade may be more amplified in adolescent and adult men also affected by acne because they share a similar pathway. Treatment of both the seborrheic dermatitis and the acne is an important therapeutic consideration to diminish overstimulation of this inflammatory cascade shared by these 2 microorganisms. However, more controlled trials examining these cohorts are needed to solidify this association.

Finally, some food for thought in regard to diet and acne: whey. The whey protein supplement market has doubled since 2007 with annual sales of $396 million last year. As of 2012, 1 in 10 men were using sports supplements at least once a week.[17] Whey protein, which has been linked to an increase in insulin growthlike factor-1, stimulates sterol response binding protein-1 that can stimulate sebaceous gland lipogenesis, comedogenesis, follicular inflammation, and androgenic stimulation (see **Fig. 1**).[18–21] One case series noted improvement of acne severity with elimination of whey supplementation.[18] However, more random controlled trials are required to prove the association with acne severity; however, it is a unique consideration regarding the male acne patient population.[21]

There are several underlying conditions that may present in male patients with acne. Classical congenital adrenal hyperplasia is more commonly recognized in female patients because of noted virilization on examination. The patients also present with salt wasting soon after birth. However, there is a nonclassical form that presents later in life. Young men presenting with precocious puberty, increased axillary and pubic hair, enlarged penis, and acne before the age of 9, should trigger an evaluation for the nonclassical form of congenital adrenal hyperplasia. Hand radiographs for bone age is an appropriate screening tool.

Laboratory investigations should include moderately elevated 17-hydroxyprogesterone (17-OHP; concentration >6 nmol/L but <100 nmol/L). If basal levels of 17-OHP are normal but still clinically suspected, a corticotropin stimulation test will demonstrate elevated 17-OHP in affected patients.[22,23] Exogenous sources of virilization should also be considered, especially in patients that demonstrate normal 17-OHP, luteinizing hormone, and dehydroepiandrosterone sulfate, and elevated testosterone. Dermal conversion of testosterone is more active in young children and should be considered if a child is in close contact with an exogenous androgen.[24]

Adolescent male acne patients are more likely to present with acne fulminans generally between the ages of 13 and 22. Acne fulminans presents with acute onset of nodulocystic inflammatory lesions, fever, myalgia, arthralgia, and bone pain. Laboratory investigations demonstrate systemic involvement with leukocytosis, elevation of erythrocyte sedimentation rate, and occasionally, anemia, proteinuria, and microscopic hematuria. Bone involvement is commonly located at the sternum and clavicle but may occur at other sites. Generally, 50% of patients have lytic bone lesions. Less commonly, these patients may also present with erythema nodosum. There have been cases of acne fulminans with underlying Crohn disease, but this is rarely reported.[25] There have also been alarming accounts of anabolic androgenic steroid–induced acne fulminans.[26] Response to traditional antibiotic therapy is inadequate to control patients with acne fulminans. Initiation of oral steroid and low-dose isotretinoin over 3 to 5 months to avoid relapse is recommended. Refractory cases may respond to azathioprine or infliximab. In contrast, a similar acute onset without systemic involvement, called pseudoacne fulminans or acne fulminans sine fulminans, may be seen in male adolescents initiated on isotretinoin therapy. The entity may also be controlled with low-dose systemic corticosteroids 0.5 to 1.0 mg/kg for 4 to 6 weeks with slow taper and decrease of isotretinoin dosage to 0.5 mg/kg/d and slowly increased as steroids are tapered.[27]

It is our differences that make us stronger, and our differences will expand our knowledge of the pathogenesis of acne. Although the understanding of the mechanism for the development of acne is in its relative infancy, as the understanding of the pathogenesis of acne expands, the differences in skin physiology between the sexes may alter the manner in which male patients are approached with acne medications. These differences may also lead to the development of new innovative treatment modalities that can target these differences.

REFERENCES

1. Luebberding S, Krueger N, Kerscher M. Skin physiology in men and women: in vivo evaluation of 300 people including TEWL, SC hydration, sebum content and skin surface pH. Int J Cosmet Sci 2013; 35:477–83.

2. Yamamoto A, Takenouchi K, Ito M. Impaired water barrier function in acne vulgaris. Arch Dermatol Res 1995;287(2):214–8.

3. Del Rosso J, Levin J. The clinical relevance of maintaining the functional integrity of the stratum corneum in both healthy and disease-affected skin. J Clin Aesthet Dermatol 2011;4(9):22–42.

4. Harper J. Gender as a clinically relevant outcome variable in acne: benefits of a fixed combination clindamycin phosphate (1.2%) and benzoyl peroxide (2.5%) aqueous gel. J Drugs Dermatol 2012; 11(12):1440–5.

5. Levin J, Del Rosso J, Momin S. How much do we really know about our favorite cosmeceutical ingredients? J Clin Aesthet Dermatol 2010;3(2):22–41.

6. Youn S, Choi C, Choi J, et al. The skin surface pH and its different influence on the development of acne lesion according to gender and age. Skin Res Technol 2013;19:131–6.

7. Eichenfield L, Del Rosso J, Mancini A, et al. Evolving perspectives on the etiology and pathogenesis of acne vulgaris. J Drugs Dermatol 2015;14(3):263–8.

8. Das S, Reynolds R. Recent advances in acne pathogenesis. Am J Clin Dermatol 2014;15(6):479–88.

9. Jalian H, Liu P, Kanchanapoomi M, et al. All-trans retinoic acid shifts Propionibacterium acnes induced matrix degradation expression profile toward matrix preservation in human monocytes. J Invest Dermatol 2008;128(12):2777–82.

10. Choi J, Piao M, Lee J. Propionibacterium acnes stimulates pro-matrix metalloproteinase-2 expression through tumor necrosis-factor alpha in human dermal fibroblasts. J Invest Dermatol 2008;128(4): 846–54.

11. Tanghetti E. The role of inflammation in the pathology of acne. J Clin Aesthet Dermatol 2013;6(9): 27–35.

12. Kurokawa F, Danby W, Ju Q, et al. New developments in our understanding of acne pathogenesis and treatment. Exp Dermatol 2009;18:821–32.

13. Bergler-Czop B, Brzezinska-Wcisto L. Dermatological problems of puberty. Postepy Dermatol Alergol 2013;30(3):178–87.

14. Clavaud C, Jourdain R, Bar-Hen A, et al. Dandruff is associated with disequilibrium in the proportion of the major bacterial and fungal populations colonizing the scalp. PLoS One 2013;8(3):e58203.

15. Kistowska M, Fenini G, Jankovic D, et al. Malassezia yeast activates the NLRP3 inflammasome in antigen-presenting cells via Syk-kinase signalling. Exp Dermatol 2014;23(12):884–9.

16. Li Z, Choi D, Sohn K, et al. Propionibacterium acnes activates the NLRP3 inflammasome in human sebocytes. J Invest Dermatol 2014;134(11):2747–56.

17. Bruising: the protein-supplement industry takes a punch. The Economist 2013.

18. Silverberg N. Whey protein precipitating moderate to severe acne flares in 5 teenaged athletes. Cutis 2012;90:70–2.

19. Melnik B. Milk consumption: aggravating factor of acne and promoter of chronic diseases of Western societies. J Dtsch Dermatol Ges 2009;7:364–70.

20. Melnik B. Evidence for acne-promoting effect of milk and other insulinotropic dairy products. Nestle Nutr Workshop Ser Pediatr Program 2011;67:131–45.

21. Bronsnick T, Murzaku E, Babar K, et al. Diet in dermatology. J Am Acad Dermatol 2014 Dec;71(6): 1039.e1–12.

22. Honour J. 17-Hydroxyprogesterone in children, adolescents, and adults. Ann Clin Biochem 2014;51(4): 424–40.

23. Bree A, Siegfried E. Acne vulgaris in preadolescent children: recommendations for evaluation. Pediatr Dermatol 2014;31(1):27–32.

24. Yu Y, Punyasavatsu N, Elder D, et al. Sexual development in a two-year-old boy induced by topical exposure to testosterone. Pediatrics 1999;104:2.

25. Zaba R, Schwartz R, Jarmuda S, et al. Acne fulminans: explosive systemic form of acne. J Eur Acad Dermatol Venereol 2010;25:501–7.

26. Kraus S, Emmert S, Schon M, et al. The dark side of beauty: acne fulminans induced by anabolic steroids in a male bodybuilder. Arch Dermatol 2012; 148(10):1210–1.

27. Grando L, Leite O, Cestari T. Pseudo-acne fulminans associated with oral isotretinoin. An Bras Dermatol 2014;89(4):657–9.

Evaluation of Acne Scars
How to Assess Them and What to Tell the Patient

Douglas Fife, MD

KEYWORDS

- Acne scar • Acne • Ice pick • Rolling • Atrophic scars

KEY POINTS

- Dermatology providers should be capable of evaluating patients with acne scars and have a discussion about treatment options.
- During the history and physical examination, the morphology and severity of acne scars are assessed, as are the patient's goals for treatment.
- A treatment plan that sets appropriate expectations and includes the most effective treatments by scar morphology and severity will maximize patient satisfaction.

INTRODUCTION

Acne scarring is an unfortunate long-term complication that can affect up to 95% of patients who have acne vulgaris.[1] The prevalence of acne scarring in the general population is estimated to be 1% to 11%.[2,3] Dermatologists should not underestimate the importance of addressing the topic of acne scars with patients. Having acne scars can be emotionally distressing to patients and can affect all aspects of their lives. Indeed, acne scars have been linked to depression, suicide, anxiety, poor self-esteem, social impairment, lowered academic performance, and unemployment.[4–6] Because of the profound effect the scars can have on a patient's quality of life, dermatology providers should take the time and develop the skills to effectively evaluate acne scars and counsel patients regarding treatment.

Although scarring can occur with any type of acne,[7] early treatment of inflammatory and nodulocystic acne is the most important way to prevent acne scars. Scars that develop during a few brief years of adolescent acne persist through the rest of life, and in some cases can worsen with normal aging or photodamage.[8] Once the scars develop, treating them can be difficult, expensive, time consuming, and often incomplete. This disease is truly one in which "an ounce of prevention is worth a pound of cure."

This report covers the evaluation of the acne scar patient and the initial discussion in which a treatment plan is established and expectations are set. A comprehensive review of each acne scar procedure is beyond the scope of this work. As with any consultations, a pertinent history and physical examination is performed, followed by a thoughtful assessment and the development of a personalized treatment plan that appropriately addresses the patient's goals for improvement. The discussion is limited to the evaluation and management of atrophic acne scars. Several other works have expertly discussed the management of keloidal acne scarring.[8–11]

HISTORY

During the initial visit, a history is taken. Important parts of the history are listed in **Box 1**. First, an assessment of the status of the patient's current acne is essential. Active acne is best brought under control before any acne scar procedures are initiated. If acne has cleared recently, perceived

Surgical Dermatology & Laser Center, 6460 Medical Center Street, Suite 350, Las Vegas, NV 89148, USA
E-mail address: dfife@surgical-dermatology.com

Dermatol Clin 34 (2016) 207–213
http://dx.doi.org/10.1016/j.det.2015.11.009
0733-8635/16/$ – see front matter © 2016 Elsevier Inc. All rights reserved.

Box 1
Examples of questions in taking an acne scar history

Current acne assessment

Is your acne under control?

How long has it been clear?

What treatments are you currently on?

Patient-specific questions

What bothers you the most about your skin?

Which scars or areas of your face concern you the most?

How are the acne scars affecting your life?

Questions that may affect treatment options

Have any prior procedures been performed to treat the scars? If so assess:

Number of sessions, associated downtime, efficacy, problems healing

What are your goals for treatment?

Was Isotretinoin used to clear the acne? When was your last dose?

Have you had any darkening of your skin from acne, surgery, or injury?

Do you have any painful, thick, or itchy scars on your body?

---

injury, or surgery will help the physician evaluate the risk of postinflammatory hyperpigmentation from energy-based or surgical procedures. Any prior procedures for acne scars should be noted, including the type of procedure, associated downtime, number of sessions, any abnormal healing, and degree of improvement.

Finally, an assessment of the patient's specific goals and expectations is taken. This assessment includes the ability to tolerate pain, tolerability of downtime, and any time constraints, such as work or travel. This assessment is an important time for the provider to assess any unrealistic expectations or signs of body dysmorphic disorder, which would be contraindications to initiating treatment.

PHYSICAL EXAMINATION

The examination of the acne scar patient includes visual inspection under appropriate lighting, active palpation of the skin, and classification of types and severity of scars. Directional or overhead lighting often helps reveal the textural irregularities. A hand-held mirror allows the patient to point out specific concerns and feel like they are completely understood. Pearls for the physician examination are listed in **Box 2**.

When visually inspecting scars, the physician should look at the scar morphology. Important scar characteristics are the depth, width, margin characteristics (sharply defined, vertical shoulder vs a gently sloping shoulder), and quality of skin at the base. Scars with normal skin at the base are amenable to more treatment options, whereas scars with hypopigmented or sclerotic skin require

scars may only be red or dark purple macular dyspigmentation that often clears on its own without any intervention. Current and past treatment of acne is assessed. Most importantly, recent isotretinoin use should be noted, as this may necessitate a delay in some resurfacing procedures.

Next, the patient's specific concerns and goals should be assessed. General questions such as "What bothers you about your skin?" or "what areas or scars you are most interested in improving?" are open-ended questions that allow the patient to express his or her desires and preferences, which may guide treatment planning. Not uncommonly, a patient may be concerned about a specific scar or area of scarring that does not appear to be the most obvious to the physician. Targeting certain scars that are most concerning to the patient may increase the chance for successful treatment and patient satisfaction.

Along with addressing active acne and assessing the patient's goals, personal and family skin history should be addressed. Are there other family members with acne scars, such as a parent or sibling? A question about history of hyperpigmentation after prior acne, inflammation,

Box 2
Pearls for the physical examination

- Evaluate for active acne.
- Use directional lighting shined tangentially on the skin to highlight atrophy/textural change.
- Have a mirror for the patient to point out lesions.
- Define types of scars (ice pick, rolling, boxcar, severely atrophic/sclerotic).
- Assess color (hypopigmentation, hyperpigmentation, purple/red discoloration).
- Assess depth and width of lesions.
- Stretch skin to see if scars disappear.
- Palpate for underlying fibrosis.
- Evaluate skin type (types III–V have increased risk of PIH with most procedures).

excisional or aggressive resurfacing procedures for improvement. Total number of scars and distribution may affect treatment plan decisions. For example, having less than 5 deep ice pick acne scars might allow a patient to be treated by a single session of punch grafting or punch excision. Alternatively, a patient with more than 100 similar lesions might be approached with a series of resurfacing procedures, as performing the required number of surgical procedures might be unfeasible because of time constraints and the densely packed nature of the lesions.

Multiple acne scar classification systems have been proposed. The simplest and arguably the most practical system divides atrophic acne scars into 3 types based on morphology: ice pick, rolling, and boxcar scars (**Fig. 1**).[12] Ice pick scars have a narrow diameter, sharply defined shoulders, and deep depth. Rolling scars have a gently sloping border and are wider than they are deep (**Fig. 2**). Boxcar scars have sharp, vertical borders which drop down to a flat base and most closely resemble varicella scars. It is common for patients to have more than one type of scar. Another useful grading system proposed by Goodman and Baron[13] uses a 4-point scale grading system to stratify severity of scarring (**Box 3**).

Although atrophic scars make up most acne scar cases, hypertrophic and keloidal scarring can occur. These types of scars are most common on the lateral face, jawline, neck, chest, upper back, and shoulders. Excellent control of acne is important in preventing new keloid scars from developing. Treatment of hypertrophic scarring can include intralesional injection of triamcinolone acetonide or 5-fluorouracil solution, silicone gel sheeting, pulse dye laser, fractional ablative or nonablative laser, or surgical excision followed by radiation or prophylactic serial triamcinolone acetonide injections.

In addition to the skin topography, any discoloration is noted, including hyperpigmentation, hypopigmentation, and red or purple discoloration. The presence of hyperpigmentation, especially in a patient with type III or darker skin type, may signify a risk for transient hyperpigmentation development after excisional or resurfacing procedures. Hypopigmentation within scars is difficult to treat and often requires either excisional procedures or fractional ablative resurfacing for improvement. Red or purple discoloration is often a temporary pigment that follows the clearance of acne nodules or cyst. This type of discoloration often makes scars appear worse than they really are. Vascular laser therapy can be performed to fade the color more quickly, but patients also can be counseled to wait on treatment planning until the color improves, as a significant improvement in the appearance of scarring can be seen as the color fades.

Palpation of scars is also helpful to assess the characteristics of the dermis underneath scars. Palpable fibrosis underneath scars may indicate poor response to fillers or subcision.[14,15] Additionally, scars that are distensible and disappear with manual stretching of the skin may do well with filler procedures or with a facelift.

PATIENT DISCUSSION AND DEVELOPMENT OF TREATMENT PLAN

Before initiating a treatment plan, an in-depth discussion should take place to address the patient's goals and to set expectations. Patient-specific issues to discuss are listed in **Box 4**. The physician should emphasize to the patient the unpredictability of acne scar treatment.[14] Although many effective treatments exist, not all patients respond to a specific procedure, and there is rarely a "quick, easy, permanent fix." Usually multiple procedures are required over a period of time. In addition, more and more patients are choosing a series of gentler treatments with minimal downtime over a period of time instead of a one-time aggressive treatment with a long period of downtime.

Instead of overpromising, physicians should attempt to give realistic expectations for improvement. If a patient is well informed about the risks and likely benefits of each procedure, they are more likely to be satisfied with their treatment, even if the results are not dramatic.

Next, a tailored treatment plan should be developed, taking into consideration the patient's goals, scar types, overall severity of acne scars, and their risk factors. **Box 5** lists treatment options available

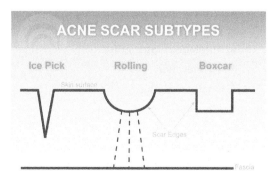

Fig. 1. Acne scar subtype classification proposed by Jacob and colleagues. (*Data from* Jacob CI, Dover JS, Kaminer MS. Acne scarring: a classification system and review of treatment options. J Am Acad Dermatol 2001;45(1):109–17.)

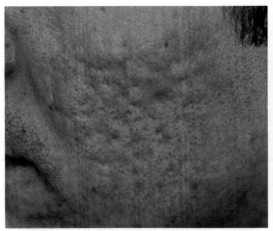 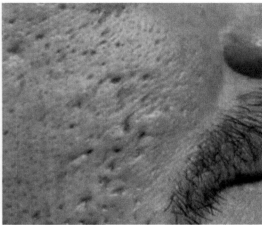

Fig. 2. Acne scar morphology. The patient on the left has rolling scars, whereas the patient on the right has ice pick scars.

Box 3
A 4-Point grading scale for acne scars

- Grade 1: Macular
  - Erythematous, hyper-, or hypopigmented marks without any textural change
- Grade 2: Mild disease
  - Mild atrophy, can be covered with makeup or facial hair
- Grade 3: Moderate disease
  - Moderate scarring, not covered by makeup but can be flattened by manual stretching of the skin
- Grade 4: Severe disease
  - Scarring not flattened with manual stretching of the skin

Data from Goodman GJ, Baron JA. Postacne scarring: a qualitative global scarring grading system. Dermatol Surg 2006;32(12):1458–66.

Box 4
Patient-specific issues to address in treatment planning

- Expectations and goals
- Financial considerations
- Time constraints
  - Important events in the distant or near future
  - Work schedule
  - Ability to tolerate downtime
- Ability of patient to tolerate discomfort

Box 5
Acne scar procedures grouped by procedure type

Acne scar treatment overview
- Resurfacing Procedures
  - Chemical peels
    - Full face
    - CROSS technique
  - Dermabrasion
  - Laser resurfacing
    - Ablative/nonablative
    - Fractional
- Lifting Procedures
  - Subcision
  - Fillers
    - Directly under scars
    - Volumizing
    - Autologous fat transfer
  - Punch elevation
- Excisional techniques
  - Punch excision
  - Elliptical excision
  - Punch grafting
- Other
  - Skin needling
  - Facelift
  - Combination techniques

to treat acne scars. Most treatment modalities can be grouped into the broad categories of lifting procedures, resurfacing procedures, and excisional procedures. Lifting procedures raise the base of the scar closer to the normal skin surface level. Resurfacing procedures cause an injury to the epidermis and superficial dermis with resulting neocollagenesis and epidermal repair. Excisional procedures completely remove scars that are deeper, sclerotic, or hypopigmented (**Fig. 3**). **Box 6** lists appropriate procedures that can be used to treat scars of a specific lesion type (eg, rolling, boxcar). If a patient has scars of varying morphologies, 2 or more different procedures may need to be selected (for example, punch excisions of ice pick scars and filler injections under soft, rolling scars).

The risks of infection, hyperpigmentation, prolonged erythema, swelling, and poor healing/scarring are present with many procedures and should be clearly explained (**Fig. 4**). It may be prudent to treat a test spot in a representative area that is in a inconspicuous location. This test may address the efficacy of a procedure, help the patient understand the downtime, and also predict the risk for side effects. Selecting the appropriate locations is important, as acne scars

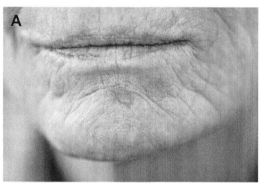

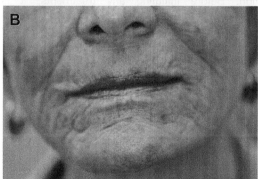

Fig. 3. Combined acne scar excision followed by fractional ablative resurfacing. (*A*) Preoperative appearance. (*B*) Final appearance.

Box 6
Procedures listed according to acne scar morphology

Macular Grade 1 scarring (redness, hypopigmented or hyperpigmented)

- No treatment (watchful waiting)
- Nonablative laser for pigment (erythema or hyperpigmentation)
- Skin needling
- Nonablative fractional resurfacing

Ice pick scars

- Punch graft or punch excision
- CROSS chemical peels

Boxcar scars

- CROSS chemical peels (for small lesions)
- Punch elevation (if good-quality skin at base of scar)
- Fractional laser therapy (ablative or nonablative)
- Fully ablative laser resurfacing
- Fractional radiofrequency
- Punch graft or punch graft (for narrow lesions)
- Elliptical excision (for larger lesions)

Rolling scars

- Filler injection immediately underneath scars
  - Temporary
    - Hyaluronic acid
    - Calcium hydroxylapatite
  - Long term to permanent
    - Poly-L-lactic acid
    - Liquid silicone polymethylmethacrylate beads
- Subcision
- Fractional laser therapy (ablative or non-ablative)
- Skin needling
- Fractional radiofrequency

Fibrotic or deep, hypopigmented scars:

- Ablative resurfacing (fractional or fully-ablative)
- Excisional techniques

Note: A combination approach in which different procedures are performed on a patient over time is usually required for optimal treatment.

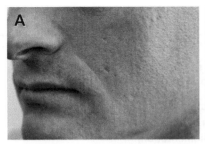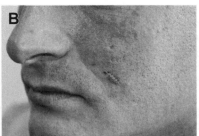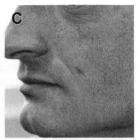

Fig. 4. Boxcar type scar (A) excised and closed with meticulous care (B). However, after 2 months the scar subsequently became hyperpigmented and depressed (C).

Box 7
Pitfalls to avoid

- Failure to set appropriate expectations
- Promising a certain level of improvement
- Failure to notice patients with unrealistic hopes or demands
- Inadequate questioning about history of postinflammatory hyperpigmentation
- Failure to assess time constraints (ie, a patient may be unhappy if there is postprocedure erythema or hyperpigmentation for an important event)
- Treating a large area with an aggressive procedure before doing a test spot.

Box 8
Treatment pearls for management

- Treat active acne before procedures for acne scars are initiated.
- Allow red/purple macular discoloration to resolve before full evaluation and treatment of atrophic scars.
- Set appropriate expectations. Emphasize that improvement is unpredictable, often multiple procedures are required. The goal should be improvement in acne scars and not total cure.
- Consider excisional techniques for fibrotic, deep, or markedly hypopigmented lesions (acne excoriee).
- In older patients with skin laxity or soft tissue atrophy consider volumizing fillers (calcium hydroxylapatite or Poly-L-lactic acid) or referral for facelift.
- Globally evaluate patent's appearance (there may be more "slam dunk" procedures such as removal of facial moles or botulinum toxin that may have more dramatic improvement).

on the chest, back, and shoulders are much more resistant to treatment than scars on the face (**Box 7**).

After combing the history, patient's goals, and physical examination and classification of scars, a treatment plan is developed (**Box 8**). Because acne scar treatments are usually not covered by insurance, a clear explanation of the costs of the entire treatment plan should be given by the physician or a staff member. Each physician has a different skill set, training, and comfort level performing acne scarring procedures. Some of the procedures can be performed by a general dermatologist and others may be performed by a procedural dermatologist who may have additional training in complicated procedures, such as punch grafting or fractional ablative laser resurfacing.

SUMMARY

Because of the high prevalence of acne vulgaris and the common associated scarring, dermatologists will inevitably be asked to provide evaluation and treatment recommendations. Having an organized approach to evaluate, counsel, and develop a tailored treatment plan will increase the chance for a positive outcome and high patient satisfaction. Before initiating any treatments, it is extremely important to understand the preferences of the patient and to set clear expectations and goals. This understanding allows the physician and the patient to form a partnership of trust as they embark on a treatment plan for treating acne scars.

REFERENCES

1. Layton AM, Henderson CA, Cunliffe WJ. A clinical evaluation of acne scarring and its incidence. Clin Exp Dermatol 1994;19:303–8.
2. Cunliffe WJ, Gould DJ. Prevalence of facial acne vulgaris in late adolescence and in adults. Br Med J 1979;1(6171):1109–10.

3. Goulden V, Stables GI, Cunliffe WJ. Prevalence of facial acne in adults. J Am Acad Dermatol 1999; 41:577–80.

4. Cotterill JA, Cunliffe WJ. Suicide in dermatologic patients. Br J Dermatol 1997;137:246–50.

5. Koo JY, Smith LL. Psychologic aspects of acne. Pediatr Dermatol 1991;8:185–8.

6. Koo J. The psychosocial impact of acne: patients' perceptions. J Am Acad Dermatol 1995;32(5 Pt 3): S26–30.

7. Goodman GJ, Baron JA. The management of postacne scarring. Dermatol Surg 2007;33(10): 1175–88.

8. Rivera AE. Acne scarring: a review and current treatment modalities. J Am Acad Dermatol 2008;59(4): 659–76.

9. Miteva M, Romanelli P. Hypertrophic and keloidal scars. In: Tosti A, Pie De Padova M, Beer K, editors. Acne scars: classification and treatment. London: Informa Healthcare; 2010. p. 11–9.

10. Shockman S, Paghdal KV, Cohen G. Medical and surgical management of keloids: a review. J Drugs Dermatol 2010;9(10):1249–57.

11. Tsao SS, Dover JS, Arndt KA, et al. Scar management: keloid, hypertrophic, atrophic, and acne scars. Semin Cutan Med Surg 2002;21(1): 46–75.

12. Jacob CI, Dover JS, Kaminer MS. Acne scarring: a classification system and review of treatment options. J Am Acad Dermatol 2001;45(1):109–17.

13. Goodman GJ, Baron JA. Postacne scarring: a qualitative global scarring grading system. Dermatol Surg 2006;32(12):1458–66.

14. Goodman GJ. Postacne Scarring: a Review of its pathophysiology and treatment. Dermatol Surg 2000;26(9):857–71.

15. Fife D. Practical evaluation and management of atrophic acne scars: tips for the general dermatologist. J Clin Aesthet Dermatol 2011;4(8):50–7.

Physical Modalities (Devices) in the Management of Acne

Mark S. Nestor, MD, PhD[a,b,*], Nicole Swenson, DO[a],
Angela Macri, DO[a]

KEYWORDS

- Acne • Treatment • Devices • Light therapy • Laser therapy • Home Devices

KEY POINTS

- *Propionibacterium acnes* is susceptible to light and laser therapies by targeting porphyrins for the improvement of acne vulgaris.
- Both visible light and laser light are effective treatments for acne.
- Patients desiring devices that can be used at home have several options for light treatment.
- Numerous clinical trials have proven both safety and efficacy for light and laser therapies for acne.

INTRODUCTION

Management of acne vulgaris is an important cornerstone of the dermatologic scope of practice. Traditional physical modalities, such as comedone extraction and solidified carbon dioxide slush, are effective in treating acne vulgaris. Comedone extraction physically removes cellular debris from the follicle, and can improve the efficacy of topical comedolytic therapy. Slush therapy, although not used routinely today, is an effective treatment of acne vulgaris.[1] Laser and light therapies and other modalities are effective treatment options for both papular, pustular, and comedonal acne. These therapies also show promise in areas where topical therapies were lacking efficacy, as in severe acne. Local side effects and adverse events are rare, and systemic side effects are absent. This paper reviews the physical properties of light and laser therapies and other available for the treatment of acne, as well as currently published clinical trials to date.

VISIBLE LIGHT PHOTOTHERAPY
Blue Light

The target of light therapy for acne vulgaris relies partly on the characteristics of *Propionibacterium acnes*, in that porphyrins produced by the bacteria absorb light in the visible spectrum. The most abundant of these is coproporphyrin III, which has peak absorption at 415 nm, and the singlet oxygen species produced by photoexcitation can eliminate *P acnes* bacteria. High-intensity blue light devices, with narrow band spectrum of 407 to 420 nm, are available for in office use. In an open-label clinical trial with a blue light device, 30 patients were treated twice weekly for a total of 5 weeks. Improvement was seen after 1 week, and at the end of treatment total acne lesions were reduced by 64%. Blue light is most effective for inflammatory acne lesions, with a reduction of papules and pustules of 69% and 73%, respectively.[2] Other studies with the high-intensity blue light have demonstrated similar efficacy in the

Disclosures: Research grants, consultant and advisory board La Lumière, LLC (Dr M.S. Nestor); No relevant disclosures (Dr N. Swenson and Dr A. Macri).
[a] Center for Clinical and Cosmetic Research, Center for Clinical Enhancement, 2925 Aventura Blvd, #205, Aventura, FL 33180, USA; [b] Department of Dermatology and Cutaneous Surgery, Department of Surgery, Division of Plastic Surgery, University of Miami Miller School of Medicine, 1600 NW 10th Ave, Miami, FL 33136, USA
* Corresponding author. Center for Clinical and Cosmetic Research, 2925 Aventura Boulevard, Suite 205, Aventura, FL 33180.
E-mail address: NestorMD@admcorp.com

Dermatol Clin 34 (2016) 215–223
http://dx.doi.org/10.1016/j.det.2015.11.003
0733-8635/16/$ – see front matter © 2016 Elsevier Inc. All rights reserved.

derm.theclinics.com

reduction of inflammatory acne lesions, and reported improvement rates range from 59% to 76%.[3,4]

Blue Light and Red Light

Combining blue light, which is effective against *P acnes*, with red light can also significantly improve acne vulgaris. Red light has an antiinflammatory effect by modulating cytokine response, and is able to penetrate deeper into the skin than blue light.[5] Various red and blue light sources have been used successfully to treat acne vulgaris. One published report of fluorescent lamps with 660 nm red light and 415 nm blue light were used by subjects with mild to moderate daily for 12 weeks, and inflammatory lesions were reduced by 75% at the end of the study, as well as a 50% reduction in noninflammatory lesions.[6] Another study included subjects with severe acne, who improved more significantly than the subjects affected mildly to moderately. A total of 24 subjects were treated with twice weekly alternating sessions of 20 minutes with 415 nm blue light and 20 minutes of 533 nm red light for a total of 8 sessions. After the 4-week treatment period, subjects were followed to 12 weeks and an overall reduction of more than 80% of both inflammatory and noninflammatory lesions.[7]

Intense Pulsed Light

The intense pulsed light (IPL) is a nonlaser device that uses flash lamps and capacitor banks to generate pulsed polychromatic, noncoherent, high-intensity light. The electrical energy is passed through xenon gas to produce light in the emission spectrum of 500 to 1200 nm.[8,9] Filters can focus the wavelength to the desired spectrum. Several mechanisms of action for IPL devices on acne have been mentioned in the literature. One mechanism involves a photodynamic effect where the absorption of ultraviolet (UV) and visible light by porphyrins in *P acnes* bacteria causes production of highly reactive free radical oxygen that subsequently kill the bacteria. Another mechanism involved is the thermolysis of blood vessels supplying the sebaceous glands. This reduces the production of sebum. Also, a photosensitizer can be applied to the skin that then accumulates in sebaceous glands, and after activated by light, can destroy the sebaceous glands.[8] Studies have shown that IPL causes an upregulation of the transforming growth factor-β1/Smad3 signaling pathway in patients with inflammatory acne.[10] ClearTouch (Radiancy, Inc, Orabgeburg, NY) was the first IPL system reported to be useful in the treatment of acne vulgaris. There are a few clinical studies on IPL devices in the treatment of acne, but they are difficult to compare because they used different devices, filters, and energy parameters. Adverse effects of IPL include pain, swelling, erythema, blistering, and crusting.[9]

Elman and colleagues[11] completed a study on 19 patients with mild to moderate acne who underwent biweekly treatments of IPL for 4 weeks. Each pulse used an average energy density of 3.5 J/cm^2, a pulse width of 35 ms, and a wavelength between 430 and 1100 nm. After the eighth treatment, noninflammatory lesions cleared 63% and inflammatory lesions cleared 50%. Acne clearance for noninflammatory and inflammatory lesions was 79% and 74%, respectively, 1 month after the last treatment and had further improvement in acne clearance at 2 months. In 2010, Kawana and colleagues[12] performed a study on 25 Japanese patients, mainly of skin phototypes III or IV, with moderate to severe acne. They were treated with IPL 5 times at wavelengths of 400 to 700 nm and 870 to 1200 nm. After the first exposure, numbers of noninflammatory and inflammatory acne lesions decreased to 36.6% and 43.0%, respectively, of their pretreatment values. After 5 treatments, they decreased to 12.9% and 11.7%, respectively, of their pretreatment values. Transient erythema with or without burning/stinging was noted in 80% of the subjects.

LASER LIGHT SOURCES
Pulsed Dye Laser

The pulsed dye laser (PDL) emits coherent yellow light in the 585 to 595 nm range.[8] Pulse durations and energy differs for different PDL devices and settings differed for different clinical studies but short pulse duration PDL may be ideal for treating acne vulgaris, as reported using the Nlight (EU-Photonics, Swansea, Wales, UK) with a 350 μs pulse.[13] PDL preferentially targets oxyhemoglobin resulting in selective photothermolysis of dilated blood vessels and causes cutaneous immunologic activation.[14] For this reason, it is particularly useful in treating inflammatory acne lesions. It is also known to stimulate dermal remodeling and collagen production, which can help to treat acne scarring.[15] PDL was originally thought to decrease *P acnes* and sebaceous gland activity; however, a study by Seaton and colleagues[16] showed that this was not the case. Instead, PDL is thought to work because of an increase in transforming growth factor-β, a potent stimulator of neocollagenesis and potent inhibitor of inflammation. Transforming growth factor-β was expressed more after PDL treatments than in IPL treatments, most likely because it has a greater photothermal effect.[17] Side effects include erythema, purpura, edema, blistering, crusting, pigmentary changes, and rarely scarring.[18]

A study by Seaton and colleagues[13] compared the effects of short pulse PDL with a sham treatment group in 41 adult patients with mild to moderate facial acne. A baseline treatment was given and patients were evaluated at 2, 4, 8, and 12 weeks after treatment. Acne severity was measured by the Leeds revised grading system. After 12 weeks, the total number of lesions decreased by 53% in the PDL group and by 9% in the sham group ($P = .023$). Inflammatory counts decreased by 49% in the PDL group and by 10% in the sham group ($P = .024$), and all treatments were well tolerated. However, in 2004 Orringer and colleagues[19] completed a study comparing PDL with a sham treatment in a split face study of 40 adult patients with facial acne and reported no differences between the PDL-treated side and the untreated side with regard to mean papule, pustule, and comedonal counts. Harto and colleagues[20] found a 57% decrease in inflammatory lesions and a 27% decrease in noninflammatory lesions after using a PDL treatment every 4 weeks for 3 times in 36 patients. When compared with topical treatments, studies showed that there were no differences in overall efficacy; however, remission of acne lesions was much higher for the PDL treated group.[21,22] Another study compared the effects of using a combination of 595-nm PDL and a 1450-nm diode laser in 15 patients with inflammatory facial acne for 3 treatments. Mean lesion counts decreased 52%, 63%, and 84% with the first, second, and third treatments, respectively, but it is difficult to say if the combination of the 2 treatment modalities was better than each on its own.[23] Jung and colleagues[17] combined a laser therapy of 585/1064-nm and compared it with just a PDL treatment alone for 3 treatment sessions at 2-week intervals. The study resulted in a decrease of total inflammatory lesions for both treatments, but the findings were not significant, and noninflammatory lesion counts were significantly decreased at week 8.

Other studies compared the effects of IPL and PDL on facial acne. In a split face study, 20 patients were treated with IPL on 1 side of the face and PDL on the other side. Both treatments were performed 4 times at 2-week intervals. Acne lesions decreased in both treatments, but inflammatory lesions showed an earlier improvement on the IPL-treated side than the PDL-treated side. However, 8 weeks after the completion of treatment, there was a rebound increase of acne observed on the IPL-treated sides. PDL showed gradual improvements, which were sustained at 8 weeks after treatment completion. Noninflammatory lesions also decreased after both treatments with the PDL-treated sides having better improvement overall. Ultimately, PDL- and IPL-treated acne effectively but PDL showed a more sustained effect.[24] Sami and colleagues[25] performed a study on 45 patients with moderate to severe acne that were randomly divided into 3 equal groups. Group 1 was treated with a PDL, group 2 was treated with IPL, and group 3 was treated with a blue–red combination LED. Results showed that the PDL was more effective and took a lesser number of treatments to reach a greater than 90% improvement than the other 2 groups. IPL was more effective than the blue–red LED treatment.

Potassium Titanyl Phosphate Laser

The potassium titanyl phosphate (KTP) laser has typically been used for vascular lesions, but has recently been used for the treatment of acne.[15] It emits pulsed green light at 532 nm. The exact mechanism of action is unclear, but is thought to cause selective photothermolysis of blood vessels and a photodynamic effect on *P acnes* and/or sebaceous glands.[15] Baugh and colleagues[26] performed a study on 26 subjects with moderate facial acne where one-half of the face was treated with 4 laser exposures with continuous contact cooling. Their results showed a mean 35% and 20% reduction at the 1- and 4-week posttreatment stages, respectively. Yilmaz and colleagues[27] studied 38 patients who underwent a once weekly or twice weekly treatment of KTP to one-half of the face. Improvements were found for both treatment groups and there was no difference found between once and twice weekly applications.

Infrared Lasers

The infrared lasers were developed originally for facial rejuvenation. They target water, which happens to be the dominant chromosphere in the sebaceous gland, thus creating a thermal injury that decreases the amount of sebum produced.[28,29] When combined with surface cooling, these lasers effectively heat the upper dermis while keeping the epidermis cool. Fluences as high as 14 J/cm^2 can be used with a cooling device.[30]

1450 nm

Friedman and colleagues[31] first reported the use of the 1450-nm diode laser in 19 patients with inflammatory facial acne. Patients underwent 1, 2, and 3 treatments at 4- to 6-week intervals and lesion counts decreased 37%, 58%, and 83%, respectively. Adverse effects were limited to transient erythema and edema. Although the pain was tolerable in this study, the 1450-nm diode laser has been known to cause considerable pain and a topical anesthetic is often recommended for use. The laser can even be used with minimal side effects in Fitzpatrick skin phototypes IV to VI. Long-term reductions in acne lesion counts can be maintained for up to 12 months after treatment.[32] One study of 38 patients reported no difference in lesion counts when performing a split face study treating 1 side of the face with the 1450-nm diode laser and the other side as a control. Both sides showed a decrease in lesion counts raising the possibility of a systemic effect of the laser.[33] A lower energy, double pass treatment with a larger 12 mm-diameter spot size has also shown to be effective for patients that complain of considerable pain.[34,35]

1540 nm

Angel and colleagues[36] performed a long-term study that used a 1540-nm erbium:glass laser with a cooling device in 25 patients with facial acne. The parameters for the laser were 3 ms, 4 pulses, 10 J/cm^2 and 2 Hz for a cumulative fluence of 40 J/cm^2. Four treatments were performed at 4-week intervals. Treatment reductions in acne lesions were 71% at 6 months, 79% at 1 year, and 73% at 2 years, and there were no side effects. Patients reported a decrease in oiliness of their skin and biopsies showed progressive rarefaction and miniaturization of sebaceous glands and pilosebaceous follicles. Another study used the 1540-nm erbium:glass laser to treat 15 patients with moderate to severe acne 4 times at 2-week intervals. At 6 months, there was a 68% improvement in patient assessments and a 78% improvement in investigator assessments. Another treatment was given 6 months after the initial course and at 9 months there was an 80% clearance compared with a 72% clearance for those who were not retreated. This study suggests the importance of maintenance therapy to prolong the lesion-free time period.[37]

1550 nm

One study used a 1550-nm (30–40 mJ) fractional erbium glass laser to treat 24 patients with 4 sessions at 2-week intervals. Patients were evaluated every 3 months for 1 year. They found a significant decrease ($P < .0001$) in the mean number of lesions at the end of the study. They also found a significant decrease in the size of the sebaceous glands using an image analyzer computer system. This finding most likely contributes to the extended lesion free period.[38]

1064 and 1320 nm

The Nd:YAG laser is another infrared laser that is typically used at a wavelength of 1064 nm for acne treatments; however, the 1320-nm laser has also been used. Orringer and colleagues[39] used the CoolTouch II 1320 nm (ICN Pharmaceuticals, Inc, Costa Mesa, CA) to conduct a split face study on 46 patients with facial acne. Three nonablative treatments were given to patients on one-half of the face. Their findings suggest that this treatment regimen may improve comedonal acne. A study used fractional 1320-nm ND:YAG laser to treat 35 patients with moderate to severe acne using 6 treatment sessions at 2-week intervals. Their results were significant and showed a 57% decrease in inflammatory lesions and a reduction of noninflammatory lesions by 35%. Chun and colleagues[40] report a case using the 1064-nm Nd:YAG laser on a 14-year-old girl with moderate to severe pustular and cystic acne. After using a topical anesthesia, they applied a topical carbon lotion to the face. They then used a Q-switched frequency-doubled Nd:YAG laser first in a quasi-long pulsed mode (a 300-μs pulse width at 1.1–1.5 J/cm^2) followed immediately by a Q-switched mode (5-nsec pulse width, 1.5–2.0 J/cm^2) using a 7-mm hand piece for both modes. Six treatments were given, 2 weeks apart. Significant improvement was noted by the fourth treatment and by the sixth treatment there was a greater than 90% improvement in inflammatory lesions. Results remained up to 8 weeks after treatment. The procedure was well-tolerated. Another study used the dual mode (quasi-long pulse and Q-switched mode) 1064-nm Nd:YAG laser with a topically applied carbon suspension in 22 subjects. They received 3 laser treatments at 2-week intervals. Results were significant showing a 59% decrease in inflammatory lesions and a 52% decrease of noninflammatory lesions on the laser treated side; however, there was a 5% increase in acne lesions on the untreated side. Mild transient erythema was the only side effect observed, but it resolved after a few hours.[41] Multiples studies have noted a significant decrease in the sebum level in patients after treatments with the Nd:YAG laser.[40,41]

Photodynamic Therapy

Photodynamic therapy (PDT) combines a photosensitizer and an activating light source to treat acne vulgaris. The 2 most common sensitizing agents are 5-aminolevulinic acid (ALA) and methyl aminolevulinate (MAL), but in the United States only ALA is available at this time. The labeled use for ALA is for the treatment of actinic keratosis, and was first described in 1990.[42] PDT with ALA can be used off label for aesthetic rejuvenation of photodamaged skin and the treatment of acne vulgaris, among other uses.[43,44] The mechanism of PDT targets both the porphyrins in *P acnes* and the sebaceous glands.[45] For the treatment of acne, the first reported pilot series of ALA was applied to the back with a 3-hour incubation and was then activated with a 550 to 700-nm red light. Patients were either treated with a single treatment or a series of 4 treatments and, when compared with red light alone, the ALA group showed a significant reduction in inflammatory lesions that was maintained until 20 weeks after the final treatment. Also, the multiple treatment regimens demonstrated significantly more improvement than the single treatment group. After treatment, erythema and edema were seen at 1 hour and resolved in all subjects. Also, a transient hyperpigmentation, crusting, and exfoliation were seen in subjects but resolved by the end of follow-up.[46] Taub[45] reported a short contact ALA-PDT treatment protocol for moderate to severe acne, in which patients were treated with 2 to 4 ALA-PDT treatments over 4 to 8 weeks with a blue visible light source. Patients had 50% to 75% improvement of inflammatory lesions after the series of treatments, and this improvement continued during the 4-month follow-up observation period. Reported side effects with ALA-PDT include mild, transient erythema and peeling.[45] ALA-PDT may be used while patients are using topical treatment regimens without an increase in adverse effects.

In addition to blue light, ALA can be activated with other light sources such as IPL and PDL. Gold and colleagues[47] reported a study that assessed the efficacy of IPL with ALA-PDT on 20 patients with moderate to severe inflammatory acne. The ALA remained in contact with skin for 1 hour before irradiation with the IPL device that emitted 430 to 1100 nm of radiation at 3 to 9 J/cm^2 fluences. Inflammatory lesions were reduced 50% at the end of a 4-week treatment period, 69% 4 weeks after the final treatment, and 72% 12 weeks after the final treatment. There were no recurrences of treated lesions and the effects were tolerated well by all patients. Rojanamatin and Choawawanich[48] reported a study that involved 14 patients with inflammatory facial acne treated with IPL on the left side and combination of IPL and topical ALA on the right side at 3- to 4-week intervals for 3 sessions. All patients revealed a reduction in number of acne lesions on both sides. The ALA-treated side showed a decrease of lesions by 87.7% at 12 weeks after the last treatment and the other side decreased 66.8%. The ALA-treated side had better

improvement overall and sustained reduction in acne lesions. One study compared the effects of IPL alone, IPL with 16% MAL, and a control. The MAL cream was applied to one-half of the face for 30 minutes before treatment. Subjects were treated 4 times at 3-week intervals. They found no differences between the treated groups and the control group with regard to the decrease in inflammatory lesion counts. However, there were significant reductions of noninflammatory lesions in the IPL with MAL group (38%) and IPL group (43%) at 12 weeks after treatment. Four patients (25%) discontinued treatment because of significant stinging, burning, and erythema after the MAL treatment.[49] ALA-PDT with activation by IPL was found to provide greater, longer lasting effects with more consistent improvements than with activation by radiofrequency combined with IPL or blue light.[50]

Pulsed dye laser is another activating light source for PDT with ALA. A study by Orringer and colleagues[51] found improvements in acne severity ratings when using ALA and PDL. The ALA was applied to the face for 60 to 90 minutes and patients received 3 PDL treatments to 1 side of the face; the other side remained untreated. The study resulted in a significant decrease in the number of inflammatory lesions. A report of complete clearance was achieved a group of 14 patients with various types of acne undergoing ALA-PDT with pulse dye laser as the activating light source. Patients received an average of 3 treatments, and were followed for 6 months with sustained improvement in the overall acne. Patients were allowed to continue topical acne products, as well as antibiotics during the study.[52]

In addition, KTP laser can be used as the light source for PDT. The effects of ALA activated by KTP laser were studied by Sadick and colleagues.[53] ALA was applied to one-half of the face and the entire face was exposed to KTP laser for 3 treatments. ALA was found to improve acne by 52% compared with 32% on the KTP only side.

In our practice, we combine microdermabrasion or photopneumatic therapy before ALA application to enhance penetration. This is followed by short pulse PDL and blue light to activate ALA. After a series of 3 treatments, patients have a significant improvement, including complete clearing in cases of severe acne with sustained results for 10 years or more after treatment.[44]

OTHER MODALITIES
Radiofrequency

Nonablative radiofrequency uses radio waves in the range of 6 to 250 MHz to heat the dermis of the skin.[54] The high temperatures are thought to kill the bacteria and reduce sebaceous glands.[55] Cryogen spray is used to help cool the epidermis. The level of penetration and energy parameters can all be modified for optimal treatment. The Thermacool device (Thermage, Inc, Hayward CA) was used in Ruiz-Espara's study of 22 subjects with moderate to severe acne. Thirteen patients were treated once and the others were treated multiple times. The average fluence per energy delivery was 72 J/cm^2. There was an excellent response seen in 18 patients, a modest response in 2 patients, and no response in 2 patients. The fluences used were well-tolerated using a topical anesthetic and there was no down time from this procedure.[56] Braun[54] reported a case where they used the combination of unipolar radiofrequency and blue light to treat severe cystic acne. The patient was treated every 2 weeks nine times with the Accent device (Alma Lasers TM, Israel). The average fluence was 100 J/cm^2. Clearance of acne lesions remained for the 8-month follow-up. The patient did not have any discomfort. A device known as the Aurora AC (Syneron Medical Ltd, Yokneam, Israel) uses the combination of pulsed light and radiofrequency. Prieto and colleagues[57] used this device to treat 32 patients twice a week for 4 weeks. They report a mean lesion count decrease of 47% after 8 treatments. Adverse effects included erythema, tingling, and burning. Biopsies were taken from 4 different patients before and after the treatment. Perifolliculitis decreased from 58% to 33%, sebaceous gland areas decreased, but heat shock protein 70 and procollagen-1 expressions did not change.

Photopneumatic Therapy

Photopneumatic system devices combine variable gentle suction pressure, approximately 3 psi, and broad wavelength visible light, from 400 to 1200 nm. In addition to removing excess sebum and comedone contents from the skin, the pneumatic action lifts the target areas closer to the light source.[58] Visible light creates singlet oxygen that react with porphyrins that reduce P acnes and damaged keratinocytes.[59] Photopneumatic devices have been studied in Fitzpatrick skin types I to IV and in mild to severe acne. A series of 11 patients with mild to moderate acne found overall significant reductions in both inflammatory and noninflammatory lesion counts after a series of 4 treatments, and reported mild treatment effects of pain, erythema, and edema after the procedure.[58] For severe acne, a series of photopneumatic treatments has been reported to improve acne significantly with reduced inflammatory

lesions.[60] A split face study is also reported in the literature, which required one-half of the face to be left untreated while the other half of the face was treated with 4 successive sessions of photopneumatic therapy. At both the end of treatment and 12 weeks after the final treatment, significant decreases in inflammatory and noninflammatory lesions were reported.[61]

Microdermabrasion

Although limited data have been published on the use of microdermabrasion to treat acne, the use of aluminum oxide microcrystals to gently exfoliate the superficial layer of the epidermis has been shown to improve the appearance of oily skin with dilated pores. After 5 sessions of microdermabrasion, 1 series reported reduced amounts perivascular inflammation and elastosis, along with increased epidermal thickness when punch biopsy specimens were examined.[62] Specifically regarding the treatment of acne, a study combining microdermabrasion and a patient's own acne treatment regimen reported a greater than 50% reduction in overall acne lesions in the majority of participants. Improvement in overall skin quality and postinflammatory pigment changes in subjects treated with microdermabrasion for acne vulgaris were reported.[63]

Ultraviolet A and Ultraviolet B

The use of UV irradiation for acne is not generally used, both because of the modest potential benefit reported in previous studies and because of the potentially carcinogenic effect of repeated exposure.[64] However, short-term narrowband UV-B has been used successfully to treat a patient with acne vulgaris during pregnancy. At a time when many topical and systemic treatments are contraindicated owing to the risk of fetal harm, UV-B treatment may be an alternative therapy.[65]

Home Use Light Devices

Both red and blue light can be used in the office to successfully treat acne vulgaris, and now devices for home use by the patient are available. In 1 study, a LED device emitting 420-nm blue light and 660-nm red light was used to treat acne vulgaris on the face twice daily by subjects for a total of 4 weeks. The subjects were monitored for an additional 8 weeks after discontinuing light treatments, and a total reduction of more than 70% inflammatory acne lesions was observed.[66] Another report of a blue light device with LEDs emitting light in the blue–violet range of 405 to 460 nm used by subjects twice weekly over a 4-week period, and complete clearance of inflammatory acne lesions occurred in 36% of patients with mild to moderate acne.[67] A 12-week randomized, controlled trial was recently completed comparing a combined 445 nm/630 nm OTC light therapy mask (illuMask®; La Lumiere, LLC, Cleveland, OH) (MASK) for the treatment of mild-to-moderate acne vulgaris. The study compared the MASK with and without topical 1% salicylic acid with retinol (MASK-SA) vs. 2.5% benzoyl peroxide (BPO). MASK-treated subjects showed a 24.4% improvement in inflammatory acne lesions (p<0.01) vs. 17.2% (p<0.05) and 22.7% (p<0.01) in BPO and MASK-SA, respectively, a 19.5% improvement in non-inflammatory lesions (p<0.001) vs. 6.3% and 4.8% for BPO and MASK-SA, respectively. Subjects in the MASK group also achieved a 19.0% improvement in the Investigator Global Acne Assessment (p<0.001) vs. 4.7% in BPO and 13.9% in MASK-SA (p<0.01). Treatments were well-tolerated overall with trends toward less early irritation in the MASK group and overall the illuMask® appears to be a safe and effective therapy for mild-to-moderate acne.[68] Other LED red and blue light devices that have been cleared by the US Food and Drug Administration for home use include brands such as Omnilux Clear-U, illuMask Acne Light Therapy, and Ocimple Light Therapy System. Also, the US Food and Drug Administration cleared LED blue light only devices that are available under the brand names DPL Nuve Blue, Quasar MD Blue for patients to use at home.[69]

SUMMARY

The variety of treatment options available for the management of acne vulgaris is significantly enhanced by laser and light therapy as well as other modalities. In comparison with topical therapies for acne, laser and light show comparable if not superior reductions in inflammatory and noninflammatory lesions. The combination of retinoid and topical antimicrobial, such as tretinoin and clindamycin, shows at least 50% improvement in overall acne appearance in 75% of patients, and marked in 50% of patients. In addition, adapalene alone will improve the number of acne lesions by 50%, and when adapalene was combined with topical benzoyl peroxide, a 61% reduction in acne lesions was reported. As with most topical acne therapies the side effects of dryness, erythema, and peeling are common.[70] The side effects of laser and light therapy are in general are in general either nonexistent or more tolerable. In addition, when compared with topical and systemic therapies, laser and light therapy without PDT for acne vulgaris is at least in theory, safe for use during pregnancy. PDT using ALA with many of the different light sources mentioned seems to be both a safe and effective for the treatment of moderate to severe acne, and light sources alone seem to be effective for mild to moderate acne. If patients prefer at home light treatments, several devices are currently available. Ultimately, combination therapy with use of topical treatment along laser and light therapy may well become the mainstay of acne therapy.

REFERENCES

1. Bolognia J, Rapini RP, Jorizzo JL. Dermatology. St Louis: Mosby; 2003. p. 542, 2180.
2. Kawada A, Aragane Y, Kameyama H, et al. Acne phototherapy with a high-intensity, enhanced, narrow-band, blue light source: an open study and in vitro investigation. J Dermatol Sci 2002;30(2): 129–35.
3. Elman M, Slatkine M, Harth Y. The effective treatment of acne vulgaris by a high-intensity, narrow band 405-420 nm light source. J Cosmet Laser Ther 2003;5(2):111–7.
4. Omi T, Bjerring P, Sato S, et al. 420 nm intense continuous light therapy for acne. J Cosmet Laser Ther 2004;6(3):156–62.
5. Lee WL, Shalita AR, Poh-Fitzpatrick MB. Comparative studies of porphyrin production in P. acnes and P. granulosum. J Bacteriol 1978;133:811–5.
6. Papageorgiou P, Katsambas A, Chu A. Phototherapy with blue (415 nm) and red (660 nm) light in the treatment of acne vulgaris. Br J Dermatol 2000; 142(5):973–8.
7. Goldberg DJ, Russell BA. Combination blue (415 nm) and red (633 nm) LED phototherapy in the treatment of mild to severe acne vulgaris. J Cosmet Laser Ther 2006;8(2):71–5.
8. Gold MH. Laser treatment of acne vulgaris. Expert Rev Anti Infect Ther 2007;5(6):1059–69.
9. Babilas P, Schreml S, Szeimies RM, et al. Intense pulsed light (IPL): a review. Lasers Surg Med 2010;42(2):93–104.
10. Ali MM, Porter RM, Gonzalez ML. Intense pulsed light enhances transforming growth factor beta1/Smad3 signaling in acne-prone skin. J Cosmet Dermatol 2013;12(3):195–203.
11. Elman M, Lask G. The role of pulsed light and heat energy (LHE) in acne clearance. J Cosmet Laser Ther 2004;6(2):91–5.
12. Kawana S, Tachihara R, Kato T, et al. Effect of smooth pulsed light at 400 to 700 and 870 to 1,200 nm for acne vulgaris in Asian skin. Dermatol Surg 2010;36(1):52–7.
13. Seaton ED, Charakida A, Mouser PE, et al. Pulsed-dye laser treatment for inflammatory acne vulgaris: randomised controlled trial. Lancet 2003; 362(9393):1347–52.

14. Omi T, Kawana S, Sato S, et al. Cutaneous immunological activation elicited by a low-fluence pulsed dye laser. Br J Dermatol 2005;153(Suppl):57–62.

15. Jih MH, Kimyai-Asadi A. Acne vulgaris: lasers, light sources and photodynamic therapy–an update 2007. Semin Plast Surg 2007;21(3):167–74.

16. Seaton ED, Mouser PE, Charakida A, et al. Investigation of the mechanism of action of nonablative pulsed-dye laser therapy in photorejuvenation and inflammatory acne vulgaris. Br J Dermatol 2006; 155(4):748–55.

17. Jung JY, Choi YS, Yoon MY, et al. Comparison of a pulsed dye laser and a combined 585/1,064-nm laser in the treatment of acne vulgaris. Dermatol Surg 2009;35(8):1181–7.

18. Levine VJ, Geronemus RG. Adverse effects associated with the 577- and 585-nm pulsed dye laser in the treatment of cutaneous vascular lesions: a study of 500 patients. J Am Acad Dermatol 1995; 32:613–7.

19. Orringer JS, Kang S, Hamilton T, et al. Treatment of acne vulgaris with a pulsed dye laser: a randomized controlled trial. JAMA 2004;291(23):2834–9.

20. Harto A, García-Morales I, Belmar P, et al. Pulsed dye laser treatment of acne. Study of clinical efficacy and mechanism of action. Actas Dermosifiliogr 2007;98(6):415–9.

21. Leheta TM. Role of the 585-nm pulsed dye laser in the treatment of acne in comparison with other topical therapeutic modalities. J Cosmet Laser Ther 2009;11(2):118–24.

22. Karsai S, Schmitt L, Raulin C. The pulsed-dye laser as an adjuvant treatment modality in acne vulgaris: a randomized controlled single-blinded trial. Br J Dermatol 2010;163(2):395–401.

23. Glaich AS, Friedman PM, Jih MH, et al. Treatment of inflammatory facial acne vulgaris with combination 595-nm pulsed-dye laser with dynamic-cooling-device and 1,450-nm diode laser. Lasers Surg Med 2006;38(3):177–80.

24. Chang SE, Ahn SJ, Rhee DY, et al. Soyun-Cho. Treatment of facial acne papules and pustules in Korean patients using an intense pulsed light device equipped with a 530- to 750-nm filter. Dermatol Surg 2007;33(6):676–9.

25. Sami NA, Attia AT, Badawi AM. Phototherapy in the treatment of acne vulgaris. J Drugs Dermatol 2008; 7(7):627–32.

26. Baugh WP, Kucaba WD. Nonablative phototherapy for acne vulgaris using the KTP 532 nm laser. Dermatol Surg 2005;31(10):1290–6.

27. Yilmaz O, Senturk N, Yuksel EP, et al. Evaluation of 532-nm KTP laser treatment efficacy on acne vulgaris with once and twice weekly applications. J Cosmet Laser Ther 2011;13(6):303–7.

28. Elman M, Lebzelter J. Light therapy in the treatment of acne vulgaris. Dermatol Surg 2004;30:139–46.

29. Paithankar DY, Ross EV, Saleh BA, et al. Acne treatment with a 1,450 nm wavelength laser and cryogen spray cooling. Lasers Surg Med 2002;31(2):106–14.

30. Rai R, Natarajan K. Laser and light based treatments of acne. Indian J Dermatol Venereol Leprol 2013; 79(3):300–9.

31. Friedman PM, Jih MH, Kimyai-Asadi A, et al. Treatment of inflammatory facial acne vulgaris with the 1450-nm diode laser: a pilot study. Dermatol Surg 2004;30(2 Pt 1):147–51.

32. Jih MH, Friedman PM, Goldberg LH, et al. The 1450-nm diode laser for facial inflammatory acne vulgaris: dose-response and 12-month follow-up study. J Am Acad Dermatol 2006;55(1):80–7.

33. Darné S, Hiscutt EL, Seukeran DC. Evaluation of the clinical efficacy of the 1,450 nm laser in acne vulgaris: a randomized split-face, investigator-blinded clinical trial. Br J Dermatol 2011;165(6):1256–62.

34. Bernstein EF. Double-pass, low-fluence laser treatment using a large spot-size 1,450 nm laser improves acne. Lasers Surg Med 2009;41(2):116–21.

35. Noborio R, Nishida E, Morita A. Clinical effect of low-energy double-pass 1450 nm laser treatment for acne in Asians. Photodermatol Photoimmunol Photomed 2009;25(1):3–7.

36. Angel S, Boineau D, Dahan S, et al. Treatment of active acne with an Er:Glass (1.54 microm) laser: a 2-year follow-up study. J Cosmet Laser Ther 2006; 8(4):171–6.

37. Bogle MA, Dover JS, Arndt KA, et al. Evaluation of the 1,540-nm Erbium:Glass laser in the treatment of inflammatory facial acne. Dermatol Surg 2007; 33(7):810–7.

38. Moneib H, Tawfik AA, Youssef SS, et al. Randomized split-face controlled study to evaluate 1550-nm fractionated erbium glass laser for treatment of acne vulgaris–an image analysis evaluation. Dermatol Surg 2014;40(11):1191–200.

39. Orringer JS, Kang S, Maier L, et al. A randomized, controlled, split-face clinical trial of 1320-nm Nd:YAG laser therapy in the treatment of acne vulgaris. Am Acad Dermatol 2007;56(3):432–8.

40. Chun SI, Calderhead RG. Carbon assisted Q-switched Nd:YAG laser treatment with two different sets of pulse width parameters offers a useful treatment modality for severe inflammatory acne: a case report. Photomed Laser Surg 2011;29(2):131–5.

41. Jung JY, Hong JS, Ahn CH, et al. Prospective randomized controlled clinical and histopathological study of acne vulgaris treated with dual mode of quasi-long pulse and Q-switched 1064-nm Nd:YAG laser assisted with a topically applied carbon suspension. J Am Acad Dermatol 2012;66(4):626–33.

42. Kennedy JC, Pottier RH, Pross DC. Photodynamic therapy with endogenous protoporphyrin IX: basic principles and present clinical experience. J Photochem Photobiol B 1990;6:143–8.

43. Gold M, Bradshaw VL, Boring MM. Split-face comparison of photodynamic therapy with 5-aminolevulinic acid and intense pulsed light versus intense pulsed light alone for photodamage. Dermatol Surg 2006;32:795–801.

44. Nestor MS, Gold MH, Kauvar AN, et al. The use of photodynamic therapy in dermatology: results of a consensus conference. J Drugs Dermatol 2006; 5(2):140–54.

45. Taub A. Photodynamic therapy for the treatment of acne: a pilot study. J Drugs Dermatol 2004;3(6 Suppl):S10–4.

46. Hongcharu W, Taylor CR, Chang Y, et al. Topical ALA-photodynamic therapy for the treatment of acne vulgaris. J Invest Dermatol 2000;115(2): 183–92.

47. Gold MH, Bradshaw VL, Boring MM, et al. The use of a novel intense pulsed light and heat source and ALA-PDT in the treatment of moderate to severe inflammatory acne vulgaris. J Drugs Dermatol 2004; 3(6 Suppl):S15–9.

48. Rojanamatin J, Choawawanich P. Treatment of inflammatory facial acne vulgaris with intense pulsed light and short contact of topical 5-aminolevulinic acid: a pilot study. Dermatol Surg 2006; 32(8):991–6 [discussion: 996–7].

49. Yeung CK, Shek SY, Bjerring P, et al. A comparative study of intense pulsed light alone and its combination with photodynamic therapy for the treatment of facial acne in Asian skin. Lasers Surg Med 2007;39(1):1–6.

50. Taub AF. A comparison of intense pulsed light, combination radiofrequency and intense pulsed light, and blue light in photodynamic therapy for acne vulgaris. J Drugs Dermatol 2007;6(10):1010–6.

51. Orringer JS, Sachs DL, Bailey E, et al. Photodynamic therapy for acne vulgaris: a randomized, controlled, split-face clinical trial of topical aminolevulinic acid and pulsed dye laser therapy. J Cosmet Dermatol 2010;9(1):28–34.

52. Alexiades-Armenakas M. Long-pulsed dye laser-mediated photodynamic therapy combined with topical therapy for mild to severe comedonal, inflammatory, or cystic acne. J Drugs Dermatol 2006;5(1):45.

53. Sadick N. An open-label, split-face study comparing the safety and efficacy of levulan kerastick (aminolevulonic acid) plus a 532 nm KTP laser to a 532 nm KTP laser alone for the treatment of moderate facial acne. J Drugs Dermatol 2010;9(3):229–33.

54. Braun M. Combination of a new radiofrequency device and blue light for the treatment of acne vulgaris. J Drugs Dermatol 2007;6(8):838–40.

55. Das S, Reynolds RV. Recent advances in acne pathogenesis: implications for therapy. Am J Clin Dermatol 2014;15(6):479–88.

56. Ruiz-Esparza J, Gomez JB. Nonablative radiofrequency for active acne vulgaris: the use of deep dermal heat in the treatment of moderate to severe active acne vulgaris (thermotherapy): a report of 22 patients. Dermatol Surg 2003;29(4):333–9 [discussion: 339].

57. Prieto VG, Zhang PS, Sadick NS. Evaluation of pulsed light and radiofrequency combined for the treatment of acne vulgaris with histologic analysis of facial skin biopsies. J Cosmet Laser Ther 2005; 7(2):63–8.

58. Gold MH, Biron J. Efficacy of a novel combination of pneumatic energy and broadband light for the treatment of acne. J Drugs Dermatol 2008;7(7):639–42.

59. Holland KT, Aldana O, Bojar RA, et al. Propionibacterium acnes and acne. Dermatology 1998;196(1): 67–8.

60. Wanitphakdeedecha R, Tanzi EL, Alster TS. Photopneumatic therapy for the treatment of acne. J Drugs Dermatol 2009;8(3):239–41.

61. Lee EJ, Lim HK, Shin MK, et al. An open-label, split-face trial evaluating efficacy and safety of photopneumatic therapy for the treatment of acne. Ann Dermatol 2012;24(3):280–6.

62. Hernandez-Perez E, Ibiett EV. Gross and microscopic findings in patients undergoing microdermabrasion for facial rejuvenation. Dermatol Surg 2001;27(7):637–40.

63. Lloyd JR. The use of microdermabrasion for acne: a pilot study. Dermatol Surg 2001;27(4):329–31.

64. Charakida A, Seaton ED, Charakida M, et al. Phototherapy in the treatment of acne vulgaris: what is its role? Am J Clin Dermatol 2004;5(4):211–6.

65. Zeichner JA. Narrowband UV-B phototherapy for the treatment of acne vulgaris during pregnancy. Arch Dermatol 2011;147(5):537–9.

66. Kwon HH, Lee JB, Yoon JY, et al. The clinical and histological effect of home-use, combination blue-red LED phototherapy for mild-to-moderate acne vulgaris in Korean patients: a double-blind, randomized controlled trial. Br J Dermatol 2013;168(5):1088–94.

67. Gold MH, Biron JA, Sensing W. Clinical and usability study to determine the safety and efficacy of the Silk'n Blue Device for the treatment of mild to moderate inflammatory acne vulgaris. J Cosmet Laser Ther 2014;16(3):108–13.

68. Nestor MS, Swenson N, Macri A, et al. Efficacy and tolerability of a combined 445 nm and 630 nm OTC light therapy mask With and without topical salicylic acid vs. topical benzoyl peroxide for the treatment of mild-to-moderate acne vulgaris. J Clin Aesthet Dermatol 2015, in press.

69. Hession MT, Markova A, Graber EM. A review of hand-held, home-use cosmetic laser and light devices. Dermatol Surg 2015;41(3):307–20.

70. Thiboutot D, Gollnick H, Bettoli V, et al. New insights into the management of acne: an update from the Global Alliance to Improve Outcomes in Acne group. J Am Acad Dermatol 2009;60(5 Suppl):S1–50.

When Acne is Not Acne

James Q. Del Rosso, DO[a],*, Nanette Silverberg, MD[b],
Joshua A. Zeichner, MD[c]

KEYWORDS

- Acne • Papulopustular disorders • Inherited syndromes • Birt Hogg Dube syndrome

KEY POINTS

- Several dermatologic conditions may simulate facial acne vulgaris, including other papulopustular disorders and inherited syndromes that produce multiple facial papules that mimic comedonal acne lesions.
- When monomorphic facial lesions are present that suggest acne vulgaris, consider other conditions; acne vulgaris usually presents with lesions in different stages of evolution.
- Many genetic syndromes present with facial papular lesions that may be confused with acne vulgaris. Many of these syndromes are associated with significant systemic abnormalities.

Acne vulgaris (AV) is generally considered to be a straightforward diagnosis that is made clinically without the availability of specific diagnostic testing to confirm the diagnosis. However, there are times when certain disorders may simulate AV, which can lead to an erroneous diagnosis and improper management. Acneiform eruptions, often associated with ingestion of certain drugs and chemicals, can confound the clinician regarding AV diagnosis.[1] Many other skin disorders can mimic AV, such as multiple small epidermal cysts or deep milia, multiple osteoma cutis, multiple small adnexal neoplasms, and follicular and/or infections characterized by multiple small papules and/or pustules such as gram-positive folliculitis, gram-negative folliculitis, *Malassezia* folliculitis, keratosis pilaris, and flat warts.[1–5] We present herein an interesting case that was originally misdiagnosed as AV.

HISTORY

A 38-year-old white woman presented with a complaint of "acne that does not go away" located on her face." She stated that she has had acne for "at least 20 years" and "nothing gets rid of the

white heads." She stated that over the past decade, she had developed "red acne bumps and pus bumps" that do go away when she uses topical medications and an oral antibiotic, but come back when she stops the medication; however, the "small white bumps never change." Previous therapies have included topical benzoyl peroxide 5%–clindamycin 1% gel, tretinoin 0.05% cream, topical adapalene 0.1%, oral doxycycline, and oral minocycline.

The patient was otherwise healthy except for mild seasonal rhinitis controlled effectively with oral loratadine. Her menses are regular and she has never attempted to get pregnant and has no children. Past medical history was remarkable for a "collapsed lung" at age 36 years. She has 2 older brothers, one who had a "collapsed lung" at age 41 years and age 46 years. Her father had a history of a "cyst on his kidney" that was surgically removed at age 44 (type unknown). Her paternal uncle had a "kidney cancer" removed when he was 48 years of age.

Clinical examination revealed multiple, monomorphic, 2- to 3-mm, round, off-white indurated papules noted diffusely on the face, predominantly involving the cheeks (**Fig.** 1A). Stretching

[a] Dermatology, Touro University Nevada, 874 American Pacific Drive, Henderson, NV 89014, USA; [b] Mount Sinai St. Luke's Roosevelt Hospital Center, 1090 Amsterdam Avenue, Suite 11D, New York, NY 10025, USA; [c] Department of Dermatology, Icahn School of Medicine at Mount Sinai, 5 East 98 Street, 5th Floor, New York, NY 10029, USA
* Corresponding author.
E-mail address: jqdelrosso@yahoo.com

Dermatol Clin 34 (2016) 225–228
http://dx.doi.org/10.1016/j.det.2015.12.002
0733-8635/16/$ – see front matter © 2016 Elsevier Inc. All rights reserved.

derm.theclinics.com

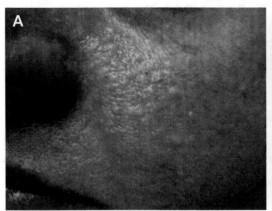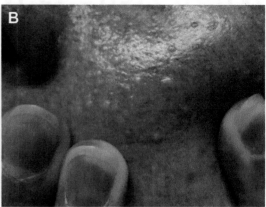

Fig. 1. (A, B) Multiple small white papules on the face suggestive of closed comedonal acne in a patient with Birt Hogg Dube syndrome. Biopsy of these papules demonstrate fibrofolliculoma/trichodiscoma histologically.

of the skin enhanced the well-defined appearance of the individual lesions (Fig. 1B). No inflammatory papules, pustules, nodules, open comedones, or acne scars were noted. No truncal involvement was noted. Differential diagnosis included comedonal AV (macrocomedones), multiple epidermal cysts, osteoma cutis, and adnexal neoplasms warranting histologic evaluation to differentiate. The monomorphic and indurated nature of the lesions raised concern regarding multiple adnexal neoplasms, which may be associated with an underlying genetic syndrome. Skin biopsy of 2 representative papules both demonstrated fibrofolliculoma. No nonfacial lesions were noted. This finding, along with the personal history of pneumothorax, and the familial history of pneumothorax and renal neoplasms including malignancy led to the diagnosis of Birt–Hogg–Dube (BHD) syndrome. Inquiry into family history revealed that her uncle with kidney malignancy underwent genetic testing which revealed an FLCN (folliculin) mutation, which confirmed the diagnosis of BHD syndrome. Although the patient was not overweight, she did report having axillary and periocular "skin tags" removed in the past, which are also a manifestation of BHD syndrome.

The patient was informed of the diagnosis and importance of further evaluation and periodic follow-up was stressed verbally and in writing, including radiographic evaluations of the chest and abdomen region to assess possible pulmonary and renal abnormalities. She delayed having the workup completely despite having good medical insurance coverage for services and stressed that her major concern was her facial appearance. Unfortunately, she did not follow-up with consultations arranged to complete her workup despite being contacted by phone and letter, and moved away from the area.

DIAGNOSIS AND MANIFESTATIONS

BHD syndrome is an autosomal-dominant, genetically inherited disorder. The major skin manifestations include a triad of fibrofolliculomas, trichodiscomas, and acrochordons, which usually manifest initially in the second to third decades of life.[6–8] Renal neoplasms, including renal malignancies, occur in 20% to 30% of cases, affecting either gender equally.[8,9] Renal malignancies, which may be solitary and unilateral or multifocal and bilateral, usually occur around 50 years of age (younger than in general population), and include diverse histologic subtypes.[8] Multiple renal cysts have also been reported, usually manifesting after the fourth decade of life.[8]

Pulmonary manifestations of BHD syndrome include lung cysts, which occur in 90% of cases, and spontaneous pneumothorax, which are seen in approximately one-fourth of cases and most often manifests after the fourth decade of life; bullous emphysema may also occur.[8,10]

CONFIRMATION OF DIAGNOSIS AND MANAGEMENT

Major criteria for diagnosis are the presence of at least 5 individual fibrofolliculoma and/or trichodiscoma lesions of adult onset noted clinically with at least 1 histologically confirmed and presence of a pathogenic FLCN germline mutation.[8,11] Other diagnostic criteria include multiple lung cysts with or without spontaneous pneumothorax, early onset renal cancer, multiple or bilateral renal cancer, or renal cancer with mixed oncocytic and chromophobe subtype histology.[8] Consultation to arrange appropriate radiologic evaluations is important both for initial evaluation and periodic surveillance.

Achrochordons may be removed easily by fine scissor excision. Treatment options for fibrofolliculomas and trichodiscomas are limited and include surgical approaches.[4,8] Laser ablation procedures

Table 1
Syndromes associated with monomorphic facial papules that may simulate acne vulgaris

Syndrome/Inheritance	Skin Findings	Other Manifestations
Brooke–Spiegler syndrome/ autosomal dominant	Trichoepitheliomas (face); cylindromas; spiradenomas	Potential for emergence of cylindrocarcinomas; carcinomatous or sarcomatous change from spiradenomas; emergence of basal cell carcinoma from trichoepitheliomas
Cowden syndrome (multiple hamartoma syndrome)/ autosomal dominant	Trichilemmomas (face); oral papillomas; acral keratosis	Breast cancer; thyroid cancer; testicular cancer; endometrial cancer; benign breast lesions (fibroadenomas, mammary hamartomas, apocrine metaplasia); uterine fibroids; mental retardation (20% of cases)
Muir–Torre syndrome/ autosomal dominant	Sebaceous neoplasms (benign and malignant) and keratoacanthomas (face)	Colorectal cancer (early onset; usually above splenic flexure); breast cancer; genitourinary cancer; stomach or small intestinal cancer
Gorlin syndrome (basal cell nevus syndrome)/ autosomal dominant	Multiple basal cell skin cancers, many on face with onset often in second or third decade of life; palmar and plantar pits	Facial dysmorphism; skeletal abnormalities (ie bifid ribs, short 4th metacarpal, digit syndactyly); ocular abnormalities; odontogenic jaw cysts; cardiac fibromas; medulloblastoma; intracranial calcifications; ovarian fibromas; lymphomesenteric cysts
Apert syndrome sporadic mutations/autosomal dominant	Severe resistant acne often widespread (face, trunk, arms, thighs, buttocks); oily skin; hyperhidrosis; interrupted eyebrows; excessive forehead wrinkling; lateral plantar hyperkeratosis; oculocutaneous hypopigmentation	Head and neck skeletal anomalies (midface hypoplasia, craniosynostosis, broad nasal bridge, cleft palate, micrognathia); low set ears; prominent forehead; vertebral fusion; symmetric syndactyly; symphalangism; mental impairment (variable)
Tuberous sclerosis (Bourneville disease; epiloia)/autosomal dominant	Angiofibromas ("adenoma sebaceum") on face; shagreen patch (connective tissue hamartoma) and ash leaf hypopigmented macules shortly after birth; periungual fibromas (Koenen tumors)	Seizures; learning disability; central nervous system tumors (giant cell astrocytoma, cortical and subcortical tubers, subependymal nodules); renal angiomyolipomas; renal cysts; polycystic kidney disease; renal cancer (rare); multiple lung cysts; cardiac rhabdomyomas; retinal phakomas (astrocytic hamartomas)

Data from Refs.[8,13–18]

have been reported.[8,12] Recurrences are common after ablative therapies. Additional management recommendations include smoking cessation and educating close family members of the diagnosis and to arrange evaluation.

BHD syndrome is only one of a variety of syndromes that can present with multiple small facial papules that can mimic AV. A selected list of these syndromes is provided in **Table 1**.

SUMMARY

Because AV is a common skin disorder encountered in clinical practice, and many dermatology practice are busy, it is important for clinicians to try and take a step back and ask themselves if they are missing something that may be critical to diagnosis and/or management for that patient. Dermatologists are human, and at times may not detect a mimicking disorder, especially those that are very rare. This case reminds us to keep in mind that a diverse group of dermatologic conditions may simulate AV.

REFERENCES

1. Momin S, Peterson A, Del Rosso JQ. A status report on drug-associated acne and acneiform eruptions. J Drugs Dermatol 2010;9(6):627–36.
2. Gjede J, Graber E. Bacterial folliculitis. In: Zeichner JA, editor. Acneiform eruptions in dermatology: a differential diagnosis. New York: Springer; 2014. p. 43–7.
3. Boni R, Nehrhoff B. Treatment of gram-negative folliculitis in patients with acne. Am J Clin Dermatol 2003;4:273–6.
4. Farris PK, Murina A. Malassezia folliculitis. In: Zeichner JA, editor. Acneiform eruptions in dermatology: a differential diagnosis. New York: Springer; 2014. p. 59–65.
5. Cunliffe WJ. Non-acne disorders of the pilosebaceous unit. In: Cunliffe WD, editor. Acne. Chicago: Dunitz-Year Book; 1989. p. 76–92.
6. Birt AR, Hogg GR, Dube WJ. Hereditary multiple fibrofolliculomas with trichodiscomas and acrochordons. Arch Dermatol 1977;113:1674–7.
7. Warwick G, Izatt L, Sawicka E. Renal cancer associated with recurrent spontaneous pneumothorax in Birt-Hogg-Dube syndrome: a case report and review of the literature. J Med Case Rep 2010;4:106.
8. Goldenberg K, Goldenberg G. Birt-Hogg-Dube syndrome. In: Zeichner JA, editor. Acneiform eruptions in dermatology: a differential diagnosis. New York: Springer; 2014. p. 183–9.
9. Pavlovich CP. Renal tumors in the Birt-Hogg-Dube syndrome. Am J Surg Pathol 2002;26(12):1542–52.
10. Ayo DS. Cystic lung disease in Birt-Hogg-Dube syndrome. Chest 2007;132(2):679–84.
11. Menko FH, van Steensel MA, Giraud S, et al, European BHD Consortium. Birt-Hogg-Dube syndrome: diagnosis and management. Lancet Oncol 2009;10(12):1199–206.
12. Gambichler T, Wolter M, Altmeyer P, et al. Treatment of Birt-Hogg-Dube syndrome with erbium:YAG laser. J Am Acad Dermatol 2000;43:856–8.
13. Glodny B, Zeichner JA. Brooke-Spiegler syndrome. In: Zeichner JA, editor. Acneiform eruptions in dermatology: a differential diagnosis. New York: Springer; 2014. p. 191–4.
14. Linkner RV, Zeichner JA. Cowden syndrome. In: Zeichner JA, editor. Acneiform eruptions in dermatology: a differential diagnosis. New York: Springer; 2014. p. 195–200.
15. Luber AJ, Zeichner JA. Muir-Torre syndrome. In: Zeichner JA, editor. Acneiform eruptions in dermatology: a differential diagnosis. New York: Springer; 2014. p. 215–20.
16. Haddican M, Spencer J, Goldenberg G. Gorlin syndrome. In: Zeichner JA, editor. Acneiform eruptions in dermatology: a differential diagnosis. New York: Springer; 2014. p. 207–14.
17. Albahrani Y, Zeichner JA. Apert syndrome. In: Zeichner JA, editor. Acneiform eruptions in dermatology: a differential diagnosis. New York: Springer; 2014. p. 179–82.
18. Pacha O, Hebert A. Tuberous sclerosis. In: Zeichner JA, editor. Acneiform eruptions in dermatology: a differential diagnosis. New York: Springer; 2014. p. 229–36.

Index

Dermatol Clin 34 (2016) 229–233
http://dx.doi.org/10.1016/S0733-8635(16)30008-0
0733-8635/16/$ – see front matter © 2016 Elsevier Inc. All rights reserved.

derm.theclinics.com

Index

Note: Page numbers of article titles are in **boldface** type.

Dermatol Clin 34 (2016) 229–233
http://dx.doi.org/10.1016/S0733-8635(16)30008-0
0733-8635/16/$ – see front matter © 2016 Elsevier Inc. All rights reserved.

derm.theclinics.com

Moving?

Make sure your subscription moves with you!

To notify us of your new address, find your **Clinics Account Number** (located on your mailing label above your name), and contact customer service at:

Email: journalscustomerservice-usa@elsevier.com

800-654-2452 (subscribers in the U.S. & Canada)
314-447-8871 (subscribers outside of the U.S. & Canada)

Fax number: 314-447-8029

Elsevier Health Sciences Division
Subscription Customer Service
3251 Riverport Lane
Maryland Heights, MO 63043

ELSEVIER

Printed and bound by CPI Group (UK) Ltd, Croydon, CR0 4YY

03/10/2024

01040384-0003